Molecular Biology and Treatment Strategies for Gliomas

Edited by Terry Lichtor

Published in London, United Kingdom

Molecular Biology and Treatment Strategies for Gliomas
http://dx.doi.org/10.5772/intechopen.110956
Edited by Terry Lichtor

Contributors
Terry Lichtor, Bingtao Tang, Edward J. Roy, Andra V. Krauze, Manendra Singh Tomar, Ashutosh Shrivastava, Bhabani Sankar Satapathy, Jnanranjan Panda, Biswabhusan Biswal, Abhishek Mishra, Snigdha Pattnaik, Pralaya Kumar Sahoo, Anshuman Gouda, Ismail Boukli Hacene, Zineb Aziza Elaouaber

First published in London, United Kingdom, 2024 by IntechOpen
IntechOpen is the global imprint of INTECHOPEN LIMITED, registered in England and Wales, registration number: 11086078, 5 Princes Gate Court, London, SW7 2QJ, United Kingdom

British Library Cataloguing-in-Publication Data
A catalogue record for this book is available from the British Library

Additional hard and PDF copies can be obtained from orders@intechopen.com

Molecular Biology and Treatment Strategies for Gliomas
Edited by Terry Lichtor
p. cm.
Print ISBN 978-1-83769-850-9
Online ISBN 978-1-83769-849-3
eBook (PDF) ISBN 978-1-83769-851-6

For EU product safety concerns:
IN TECH d.o.o., Prolaz Marije Krucifikse Kozulić 3, 51000 Rijeka, Croatia,
info@intechopen.com or visit our website at intechopen.com.

Meet the editor

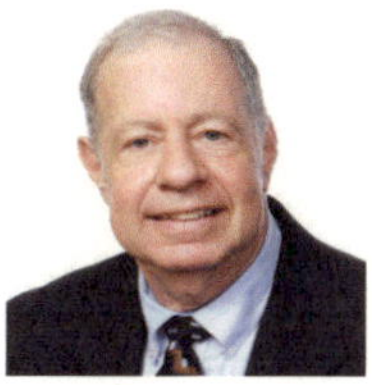

Terry Lichtor, MD, Ph.D., is a practicing neurosurgeon. He has several research interests, and his brain tumor work is largely focused on the development of a DNA vaccine for the treatment of primary and metastatic intracerebral tumors. Dr. Lichtor has shown that vaccines prepared by the transfer of DNA from the tumor into a highly immunogenic cell line can encompass the array of tumor antigens that characterize the patient population. Poorly immunogenic tumor antigens, characteristic of malignant cells, can become strongly antigenic if they are expressed by highly immunogenic cells. The introduction of the vaccine directly into the tumor bed of animals with an intracerebral tumor stimulates a systemic cellular anti-tumor immune response associated with a prolongation of survival. Hopefully, this vaccine strategy will be efficacious in the treatment of patients with brain tumors. Dr. Lichtor is a member of the American College of Surgeons and the neurosurgery faculty at Rush University Medical Center, Chicago, Illinois, USA.

Contents

Preface IX

Section 1
Development of Novel Potential Glioma Treatment Options 1

Chapter 1 3
Development of a Brain Tumor Vaccine
by Terry Lichtor, Bingtao Tang and Edward J. Roy

Chapter 2 23
Attributing Meaning to Molecular Interaction Networks by Leveraging Clinical and Omic Data: The Missing Link between Tumor Biology and Treatment Strategies in Glioma
by Andra V. Krauze

Chapter 3 39
Role of miRNA in Glioma Pathogenesis, Diagnosis, and Therapeutic Outcomes
by Manendra Singh Tomar and Ashutosh Shrivastava

Chapter 4 59
Magnetic Nanocarrier Based Drug Targeting: Emerging Trend for the Treatment of Glioma
by Bhabani Sankar Satapathy, Jnanranjan Panda, Biswabhusan Biswal, Abhishek Mishra, Snigdha Pattnaik, Pralaya Kumar Sahoo and Anshuman Gouda

Section 2
4D MRI Glioma Tumor Classification 79

Chapter 5 81
Deep Learning for Computer-Aided Diagnosis (CAD) of Brain Diseases Four-Dimensional Magnetic Resonance Imaging (4D MRI Classification) from Glioma Tumor
by Ismail Boukli Hacene and Zineb Aziza Elaouaber

Preface

Although technical advances have resulted in marked improvements in the ability to diagnose and surgically treat primary and metastatic brain tumors, the incidence and mortality rates of these tumors are increasing. The present standard treatment modalities following surgical resection, including cranial irradiation and systemic or local chemotherapy, each have limited efficacy and serious adverse side effects. Furthermore, the relatively few long-term survivors are inevitably left with cognitive deficits and other disabilities. The difficulties in treating malignant gliomas can be attributed to several factors. Glial tumors are inherently resistant to radiation and standard cytotoxic chemotherapies. The existence of blood–brain and blood–tumor barriers impedes drug delivery to the tumor and adjacent brain infiltrated with the tumor. In addition, the low therapeutic index between tumor sensitivity and toxicity to the normal brain severely limits the ability to systemically deliver therapeutic doses of drugs or radiation therapy to the tumor. New treatment strategies for the management of patients with these tumors are urgently needed.

This book describes some improvements in the surgical management of gliomas, including segmentation of brain MRI images using 4D MRI volumes to help with the diagnosis and monitoring of patients. Another novel topic reviewed in this book involves the applications of photosensitizers and their efficacy in the generation of anti-tumor responses in photodynamic therapy. The application of nanoparticles and their ability to deliver drugs to the tumor site with a reduction in systemic toxicity is another therapy in development that is discussed in this volume. The book also reviews novel approaches involving the development of the use of microRNAs, which are non-coding RNAs that can be used as tumor suppressors that potentially can be developed to control the growth of gliomas. Another study involves an understanding of the large number of molecular interactions of signals in gliomas, which should lead to biomarkers of potential importance that could be manipulated in the development of clinical trials. Molecular networks need to be better understood for the development of therapeutic strategies. Finally, the book discusses immunotherapeutic strategies, which involve either poxviruses engineered to secrete IL-15 or IL-2 secreting fibroblasts transfected with tumor DNA, that can be potentially useful in treating brain tumors. The stimulation of the immune system to selectively attack malignant cells should lead to the prolongation of survival of patients with brain tumors without a decline in cognitive functions or other side effects. Hopefully, this new information will lead to improved and efficacious treatment strategies for these challenging tumors.

Terry Lichtor, MD, Ph.D.
Department of Neurosurgery,
Rush University Medical Center,
Chicago, Illinois, USA

Section 1

Development of Novel Potential Glioma Treatment Options

Chapter 1

Development of a Brain Tumor Vaccine

Terry Lichtor, Bingtao Tang and Edward J. Roy

Abstract

Glioma is a malignant brain tumor associated with a poor outcome. Attempts at surgical removal of the tumor are the first approach. Additional necessary treatment strategies including cranial irradiation and systemic or local chemotherapy each have serious side effects and provide relatively minimal survival benefits. Antigenic differences between normal and malignant cells of the cancer patient form the rationale for clinical immunotherapeutic strategies. Cytokines such as IL-15 or IL-2 that stimulate an antitumor immune response have been shown to have a particularly high potential for use in immunotherapy against various tumors. In this chapter studies with either a poxvirus genetically engineered to secrete IL-15 or allogeneic fibroblasts engineered to secrete IL-2 are shown to be an effective treatment strategy in prolonging survival in mice with malignant intracerebral tumors upon injection of the treatment cells into the brain. Future studies with these treatment strategies in patients with intracerebral tumors are urgently needed.

Keywords: immunotherapy, IL-2, IL-15, brain tumors, prolonged survival

1. Introduction

1.1 Limitation of current brain tumor treatments

Some increase in the ability to diagnose and surgically treat primary brain tumors has been achieved, although the mortality and overall survival of patients with these tumors has not improved over many years [1]. The present standard treatment modalities following surgery to remove the tumors followed by radiation therapy and chemotherapy each have significant side effects. The long-term survivors are few and often left with cognitive deficits and other disabilities [2, 3]. Gliomas are resistant to adjuvant treatments including radiation and cytotoxic chemotherapies making it difficult to treat these tumors [4, 5]. Novel therapies are urgently needed.

1.2 Principles of brain tumor immunology

Antigenic differences between normal and malignant cells of the cancer patient form the rationale for clinical immunotherapeutic strategies. Several different strategies have been attempted to enhance the anti-tumor immune responses in mice and patients with intracerebral neoplasms. Immunization with dendritic cells provided with derivatives of tumor cells or transfected with tumor-RNA can result in the development of immune responses against antigens expressed by the tumor cells [6, 7]. Immunization in patients with dendritic cells transfected with mRNA from malignant glioma has been found to elicit tumor-specific $CD8^{+}$ cytotoxic T-lymphocyte (CTL) responses against the patient's tumor [8]. Novel and more specific targets such as glioma stem cells have been shown to improve the success of dendritic cell immunotherapy [9]. Although results of dendritic cell immunotherapy have demonstrated promise in animal models, clinical trials have documented only short benefits in a limited number of patients [10].

Another strategy involves a vaccine prepared by transfer of a cDNA expression library derived from tumor cells into an allogeneic mouse fibroblast cell line expressing a cytokine such as IL-2, which appears to have great potential in the development of an antitumor immune response in the treatment of an intracerebral tumor in mouse models [11]. Upon transfer of the cDNA-expression library from the tumor cells into a highly immunogenic fibroblast cell line, genes specifying an array of tumor antigens are expressed. The transferred DNA integrates into the genome of the recipient cells and replicates as the cells divide. The transfected fibroblasts can be expanded to obtain quantities for repeated immunizations of the patient. This strategy should be capable of inducing immunity to a broad array of tumor antigens that characterize the patient's tumor. Enough DNA to prepare the vaccine can be obtained from small amounts of tumor tissue (4 mm), enabling treatment at an early stage of the disease.

In many aggressive tumors, such as gliomas, progression is enhanced by local immunosuppression associated with the accumulation of regulatory T-cells (Treg) and myeloid-derived suppressor cells (MDSC) [12]. The lack of response to treatment in glioma patients may be attributed to the immunosuppressive T-cells that normally prevent autoimmunity when the human immune response is evoked [13]. Various cytokines including interleukin-10 and transforming growth factor-β have been implicated in the stimulation of Tregs. The targeting of immune checkpoints that regulate the immune system is emerging as a potent and viable cancer therapy [14]. Immunosuppressive mediators such as IL-10, TGF-β and prostaglandin can inhibit the function of the immune system and promote the growth of tumors [15]. Reversing the immunosuppressive tumor microenvironment is one of the keys to the success of tumor treatment.

There are several immunomodulatory cytokines including IL-2, IL-4, IL-7, IL-9, IL-15 and IL-21 which belong to the family of four α-helix bundle cytokines [16]. The development of IL-2 has been a sentinel force in the development of immunotherapy in cancer [17]. However, the use of IL-2 is limited by toxicity and the expansion of regulatory T-cells. These limitations can be overcome with the use of other T-cell stimulatory agents such as IL-15 which also has been in clinical development. IL-15 has been shown to have a particularly high potential for use in immunotherapy against various tumors [18]. Furthermore, IL-15 unlike IL-2 does not contribute to the maintenance of regulatory T-cells [19].

A variety of tumor vaccination strategies have been attempted including modification of neoplastic cells to stimulate anti-tumor immune responses. Immunization with tumor cells modified to secrete cytokines such as IL-2, IFN-γ and GM-CSF has resulted in the development of MHC-restricted anti-tumor immune responses in animal models [20–28]. Tumor regression has been documented in experimental animals receiving immunotherapy alone, which suggests that this treatment strategy may be effective.

1.3 Potential applications of oncolytic viruses in brain tumor therapy

An oncolytic virus is a type of virus, either engineered or in nature, which may infect and lyse tumor cells but not affect normal cells [29]. There are many oncolytic viruses which include herpes simplex virus (HSV), adenovirus, reovirus, poliovirus (PV), vaccinia virus (VV), myxoma virus (vMyx), measles virus, vesicular stomatitis virus (VSV) and newcastle disease virus [30]. There are multiple potential mechanisms contributing to the selectivity of oncolytic viruses for tumor cells over normal cells. First, viruses can enter tumor cells by binding with certain receptors which are overexpressed on the tumor cells' surface. For instance, HSV binds herpes virus entry mediator (HVEM) or nectin-1, VV binds glycosaminoglycans (GAGs) and VSV binds low-density lipoprotein receptor (LDLR) to enter host cells.

Second, some of the hyper-activated signaling pathways in tumor cells over normal cells may facilitate virus infection. Hyper-activation of AKT (serine/threonine kinase) is commonly found in most cancer cells which is a requirement for vMyx infection [31, 32]. EGFR activation, common in cancer cells, contributes to a productive infection by the attenuated vaccinia virus JX-594 [33]. Third, deficiency of tumor cells to Type I interferon responses minimize the anti-viral immune responses allowing oncolytic viruses replication [34, 35]. Fourth, dysfunction of tumor suppressor genes, such as p53, ataxia telangiectasia (ATM) and retinoblastoma protein (Rb) can potentially compromise cellular antiviral activity by accumulating genomic instability and blocking the apoptotic response [36] which contributes to the permissiveness of cancer cells.

Once oncolytic viruses infect tumor cells, they may contribute to the anti-tumor response by a direct cytotoxic effect on tumor cells and consequent release of tumor antigens which could stimulate anti-tumor immune responses [37]. When the virus is engineered to express an immunostimulatory cytokine [38], it becomes a vector for local expression of potent immune-activating agents, attracting immune cells into the tumor microenvironment (TME) while limiting inflammation that systemic delivery of the cytokine might produce.

Many oncolytic viruses have already been tested in several preclinical and clinical trials. T-VEC (also known as Talimogene laherparepvec or OncoVEX^{GM-CSF}) is the first oncolytic virus approved for the treatment of advanced melanoma by the U.S. Food and Drug Administration (FDA) in 2015 [39]. T-VEC is an engineered oncolytic herpes simplex virus type 1 (HSV-1), whose neurovirulence factor ICP34.5 is replaced by the gene of human granulocyte-macrophage colony-stimulating factor (hGM-CSF) and the viral ICP47 gene is deleted [40], to prevent neuronal involvement [41] and enhance anti-tumor efficacy. An OPTiM phase III clinical trial showed the efficacy of T-VEC to target patients with early metastatic melanoma (stage IIIB/C-IVM1a) [42]. It also showed enhanced antitumor activity when T-VEC was combined with pembrolizumab (anti-programmed death-ligand 1 antibody; PD-1 blockade) in a phase II clinical trial [43]. In addition, G47Δ, a triple-mutated, third-generation oncolytic HSV-1 [44] was demonstrated with a high safety profile and high anti-tumor efficacy (1-year survival rate 92.3 versus 15%) when targeting human glioblastoma in a phase II clinical trial [45].

Poliovirus is another potential candidate for oncolytic virotherapy. The recombinant nonpathogenic polio–rhinovirus chimera (PVSRIPO) is a neuro-attenuated recombinant poliovirus (Sabin vaccine strains), whose internal ribosomal entry site (IRES) was replaced with human rhinovirus type 2 (HRV2) [46]. The result from a phase I clinical trial, where 61 patients with recurrent World Health Organization

(WHO) grade IV malignant glioma were intratumorally infused with PVSRIPO, confirmed the safety of PVSRIPO used in the brain and showed significantly higher survival rate at 24 and 36 months after virus infusion [47]. Studies also showed that PVSRIPO has the potential to show therapeutic effects on breast cancer, prostate cancer [48] and neuroblastoma [49].

Poxvirus, a group of large, enveloped DNA viruses associated with diseases that generate poxes in the skin, can also be a good choice for oncolytic virotherapy since the entire replication of poxvirus happens in viral factories within the cytoplasm of infected cells with no integration of viral DNA into host genome which is safe for host cells [50]. Poxviruses can take multiple large foreign genes into their genomes [51] which supports the feasibility of further arm poxviruses (e.g., adding genes of tumor antigen or immune-enhancing cytokines to poxviruses). vvDD vaccinia virus is a new strain of poxvirus which was attenuated by double deletion of thymidine kinase and vaccinia growth factor. A preclinical study showed great anti-tumor efficacy when mice bearing MC38 colon cancer or ID8 ovarian cancer were treated with IL15 armed vvDD vaccinia virus. In addition, when combined with PD-1 blockade, IL15 armed vvDD vaccinia virus leads to dramatic tumor regression [52]. It has been reported that IL15 armed myxoma virus (another poxvirus) cured 83% of mice bearing orthotopic glioma when combined with adoptive T-cell therapy, rapamycin and celecoxib [53].

Despite the promising results, some concerns still need attention when using oncolytic viruses. One major concern for oncolytic virotherapy is the safety issue of the oncolytic virus. For example, vvDD vaccinia virus which has undergone two phase I clinical trials and has been found safe in humans [54, 55] can still be fatal for hosts if it accidentally enters the cerebral lateral ventricle [56]. Therefore, it is essential to study the safety profile of the oncolytic virus thoroughly before moving to clinical trials. Another concern is the development of the anti-viral immune responses mediated by neutralizing antibodies [57] and immune cells such as macrophages [58] and natural killer [59] (NK) cells which can diminish the ability of the virus to enhance anti-tumor immunity.

2. Pre-clinical experimental findings

2.1 Survival of mice with intracerebral glioma upon treatment with fibroblasts engineered to secrete cytokines

Gl261 cells are a glioma cell line of C57Bl/6 mouse origin ($H\text{-}2^b$). LM fibroblasts are derived from C3H/He mice and express $H\text{-}2^k$ determinants. The potential development of an antitumor immune response was explored using fibroblasts engineered to secrete either IL-2 or IL-2 and interferon- injected into the brain in mice with an intracerebral (i.c.) glioma [60]. Glioma cells were mixed with cells secreting one or two of the cytokines of interest and subsequently were injected i.c. into the right frontal lobe of C57BL/6 mice which are syngeneic with G1261 cells. The results (**Figure 1**) demonstrate that IL-2-secreting fibroblasts were capable of prolonging survival in mice with a right frontal glioma upon i.c. injection of the treatment cells ($P < 0.025$). The results were more dramatic upon i.c. injection of mice with glioma treated with LM-IL-2/interferon- double cytokine-secreting cells ($P < 0.005$). The i.c. injection of mice with equivalent numbers of LM-IL-2 cells without tumors lived many months and did not demonstrate ill effects or neurologic deficit.

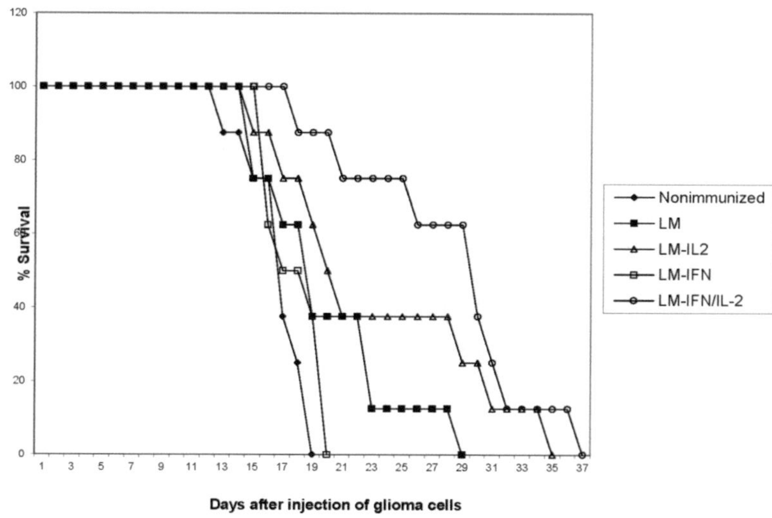

Figure 1.
Treatment of intracerebral glioma in C57Bl/6 mice by immunization with allogeneic cytokine-secreting fibroblasts. The C57Bl/6 mice (8 per group) were injected i.c. with a mixture of 10^6 cells of one of the cell types and 10^5 Gl261 glioma cells. Gl261 is a malignant glial tumor syngeneic in C57Bl/6 mice. The median lengths of survival were as follows (in days): Mice with nonimmunized glioma cells, 16.9 1.9; glioma plus LM cells, 20.0 4.5; glioma plus LM-IL-2 cells, 23.4 6.8; glioma plus LM-IFN-(cells, 18.0 1.8; glioma plus LM-IL-2/IFN-γ cells, 28.1 5.8. Probability values were: Nonimmunized vs. LM-IL-2, $p < 0.025$; nonimmunized or LM vs. LM-IL-2/IFN-γ, $p < 0.005$; LM-IL-2 vs. LM-IL-2/IFN-γ, $p < 0.05$.

2.2 Immunocytotoxic studies from spleen cells with mice treated with allogeneic cytokine-secreting fibroblasts

A chromium release assay was used to determine the reactivity of spleen cells from the immunized mice to chromium-labeled Gl261 glioma cells. The results [60] demonstrate a significantly elevated chromium release when spleen cells from the mice with i.c. Gl261 cells treated with cytokine-secreting fibroblasts were co-incubated with chromium-labeled Gl261 cells. This data documents the development of a systemic anti-tumor immune response in the mice injected with the cytokine-secreting cells. Antibody depletion studies reveal that the antitumor immunity was mediated both by $CD8^+$ and NK/LAK cells.

2.3 Treatment of glioma in mice treated with IL-15 secreting cells

Two oncolytic poxviruses, vvDD vaccina virus and myxoma virus, were engineered to express the fusion protein IL15Ra-IL15 (53). Viral gene expression was confirmed in the murine glioma by staining for M-T7 (a myxoma-encoded protein) and IL-15 (**Figure 2A**). Mice with glioma were treated with either of these two viruses supplemented by rapamycin, celecoxib and adoptive T-cell therapy (tumor-specific $CD8^+$ T-cells). Rapamycin was used to enhance the spread and replication of oncolytic viruses [61–63], while celecoxib should reduce the immunosuppressive tumor microenvironment by inhibiting the production of prostaglandins (mainly PGE2) [15, 64]. Direct injection of vvDD-IL15-Rα into the lateral cerebral ventricles was uniformly fatal, whereas mice that received intracerebral vMyx-IL15Rα-tdTr injection recovered from the virus infection [56]. This suggests that vvDD vaccinia virus may not be a safe choice to treat tumors inside of the brain, whereas myxoma virus could be a potential

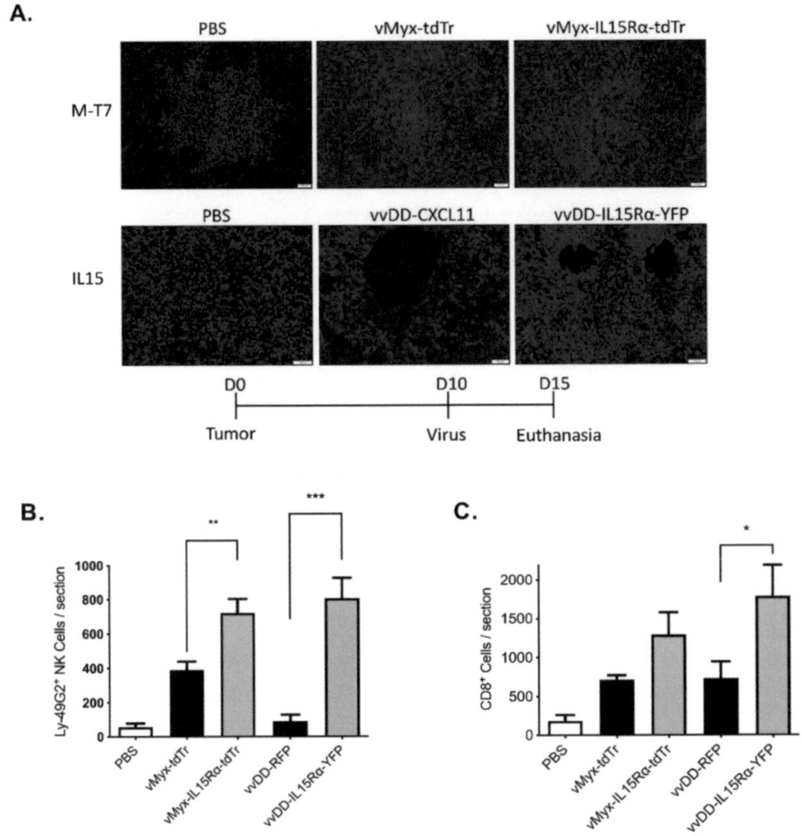

Figure 2.
In vivo characterization of vMyx-tdTr, vMyx-IL15Rα-tdTr, vvDD-RFP, vvDD-CXCL11 and vvDD-IL15Rα-YFP. C57BL/6J mice were implanted with GL261 NS cells i.c. followed 10 days later by injection with PBS, vMyx-tdTr, vMyx-IL15Rα-tdTr, vvDD-CXCL11 or vvDD-IL15Rα-YFP. Alternatively, mice received i.c. injections of vMyx-tdTr, vMyx-IL15Rα-tdTr, vvDD-RFP or vvDD-IL15Rα-YFP. (n = (2 × 10^6 pfu intratumoral). Mice were euthanized 5 days after the virus treatment and tumor sections were analyzed for the presence of the viruses, IL15, NK cells and $CD8^+$ T-cells by immunostaining for M-T7 (a myxoma-encoded protein), IL15, Ly-49G2 (4D11 antibody) for NK cells and CD8, respectively. Representative tumor sections are shown. **A.** *Staining for M-T7 or IL15 expression in tumors. Scale bar = 200 microns.* **B.** *Number of Ly-49G2$^+$ NK cells per tumor section for each condition, mean values and SEM are shown. One-way ANOVA showed a significant increase in NK cell accumulation in vMyx-IL15Rα-tdTr or vvDD-IL15Rα-YFP treated tumors compared to vMyx-tdTr or vvDD-RFP treatments (** $p < 0.01$; *** $p < 0.001$).* **C.** *Number of $CD8^+$ cells per tumor section for each condition, mean values and SEM are shown. One-way ANOVA showed a significant increase in $CD8^+$ cell accumulation in vvDD-IL15Rα-YFP treated tumors compared to vvDD-RFP treatment (* $p < 0.05$).*

alternative. Mice that received intracerebral vMyx-IL15Rα-tdTr injection recovered from the virus infection [56].

To explore the anti-tumor efficacy of myxoma virus expressing IL15, the combination treatment (vMyx-IL15Rα-tdTr, rapamycin, celecoxib and adoptive T-cell transfer therapy) was applied to tumor-bearing mice. An increased number of infiltrating NK and $CD8^+$ T-cells was detected in the tumor specimens (**Figure 2B,C**) indicating that the IL15Rα-IL15 fusion protein is biologically functional and could attract NK and $CD8^+$ T-cells into the tumor site. The prolongation of survival ($P < 0.01$ compared to untreated animals or animals that did not receive Celecoxib) (**Figure 3**) indicated that myxoma virus (vMyx-IL15Rα-tdTr) supplemented by rapamycin and the

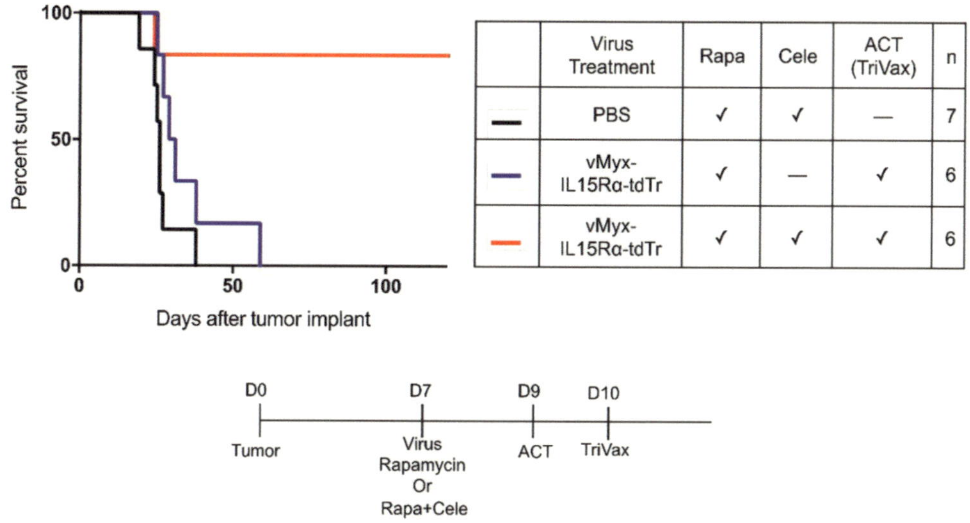

	Virus Treatment	Rapa	Cele	ACT (TriVax)	n
— (black)	PBS	✓	✓	—	7
— (purple)	vMyx-IL15Rα-tdTr	✓	—	✓	6
— (orange)	vMyx-IL15Rα-tdTr	✓	✓	✓	6

Figure 3.
The therapeutic effect of the full combination treatment using vMyx-IL15Rα-tdTr. Survival of tumor-bearing mice treated with intratumoral vMyx-IL15Rα-tdTr virus injection, rapamycin and celecoxib, adoptive transfer of CD8⁺ T-cells and TriVax booster. Mice received tumor on day 0, 1 μL vMyx-IL15Rα-tdTr virus (2 x 10^6 pfu) or PBS injection, rapamycin with or without celecoxib on day 7 (medication treatment continued until day 73), adoptive transfer of $CD8^+$ T-cells on day 9, TriVax booster on day 10. Mice that received the full combination treatment survived longer compared to other groups. $p < 0.05$ for each comparison.

prostaglandin inhibitor celecoxib could provide a safe and effective anti-tumor treatment in mice with intracerebral glioma upon injection of the treatment cells into the brain or lateral ventricles. The efficacy of this novel combination treatment strategy in glioma-bearing mice following tumor resection is being explored [65].

2.4 Immunization with allogeneic cytokine-secreting fibroblasts transfected with DNA from breast cancer in treatment of C3H mice with intracerebral breast cancer

A tumor vaccine was constructed by transfer of DNA from a breast cancer cell line (SB-5b) that arose in C3H mice ($H\text{-}2^K$) into cytokine-secreting mouse fibroblasts ($H\text{-}2^K$). The application of these cells as a potential treatment of an intracerebral breast neoplasm arising in C3H mice was investigated. The cells were modified to express $H\text{-}2K^b$ determinants, and this should also ensure rejection. Studies with these cells revealed that there was a prolongation of survival (**Figure 4**) in C3H mice with intracerebral breast cancer upon treatment by immunization with fibroblasts secreting either IL-2 or GM-CSF transfected with DNA from the same spontaneous breast neoplasm ($P < 0.05$) [66].

2.5 The proportion of splenic T-cells reactive with SB-5b tumor cells in mice immunized with transfected cytokine-secreting fibroblasts

An ELISPOT-IFN- assay was used to estimate the development of splenic T-cells reactive with SB-5b cells in mice immunized with transfected fibroblasts modified to secrete IL-2 or GM-CSF. The assay was performed 6 weeks after the i.c. injection of the mixture of SB-5b cells and the transfected fibroblasts. The findings in these

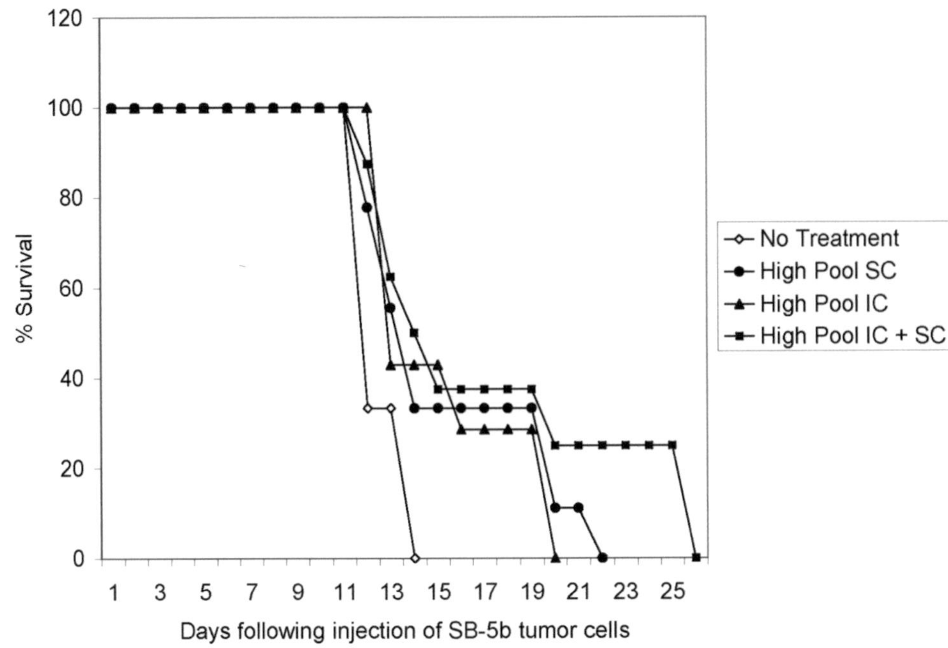

Figure 4.
Treatment of C3H/He mice with intracerebral SB-5b breast carcinoma with mice immunized with cytokine-secreting allogeneic fibroblasts transfected with DNA from a spontaneous breast neoplasm (SB-5b). C3H/He mice (nine animals/group) were injected with a mixture of 1.0 X 10^4 *SB-5b cells and 1.0 X* 10^6 *cytokine-secreting fibroblasts transfected with tumor DNA or with an equivalent number of non-secreting cells transfected with tumor DNA (*LMK^b*/SB5b). Mean survival time (MST) in days: Media control, 23.0 1.9;* LMK^b*/SB5b, 27.3 6.3;* LMK^b*GMCSF/SB5b, 30.0 9.5;* LMK^b*IL-2/SB5b, 36.6 7.0;* LMK^b*IL-18/SB5b, 28.4 4.8. Probability values were as follows:* LMK^b*IL-2/SB5b vs.* LMK^b*/SB5b or media control,* $P < 0.005$*;* LMK^b*IL-2/SB5b vs.* LMK^b*IL-18/SB5b,* $P < 0.025$*;* LMK^b*IL-2/SB5b vs.* LMK^b*GMCSF/SB5b,* $P < 0.05$*;* LMK^b*GMCSF/SB5b vs. media control,* $P < 0.05$*.*

studies revealed that the highest proportion of T-cells reactive with SB-5b cells was in surviving mice injected with fibroblasts modified to secrete IL-2 (**Figure 5A**). Lesser numbers of spots were found in T-cells from mice injected with SB-5b cells and non-secreting transfected fibroblasts or SB-5b cells and transfected fibroblasts modified to secrete GM-CSF.

In additional experiments, animals with i.c. breast cancer were treated i.c. with LMK^bIL-2/SB5b cells. An ELISPOT assay was done after 2 weeks using the spleen cells to detect IFN- secretion in the presence or absence of SB-5b tumor cells and antibodies against various T-cell subsets. These studies revealed that $CD4^+$, $CD8^+$ and NK/LAK cells were responsible for the antitumor immune response (**Figure 5B**). The overall P-value between the unstimulated vs. the tumor cell stimulated group is $P < 0.001$.

2.6 Development of an enrichment strategy for a more potent vaccine

A strategy was developed to enrich the vaccine for efficacy by identifying cell populations that were the most highly immunogenic [11]. Populations with higher numbers of immunogenic cytokine-secreting cells transfected with tumor DNA were identified by their stronger antitumor immune response against SB5b cells in C3H/He mice. Two sub-pools that stimulated immunity to the greatest (immuno^{high} pool) and least (immuno^{low} pool) after three rounds of enrichment were identified and used in further studies.

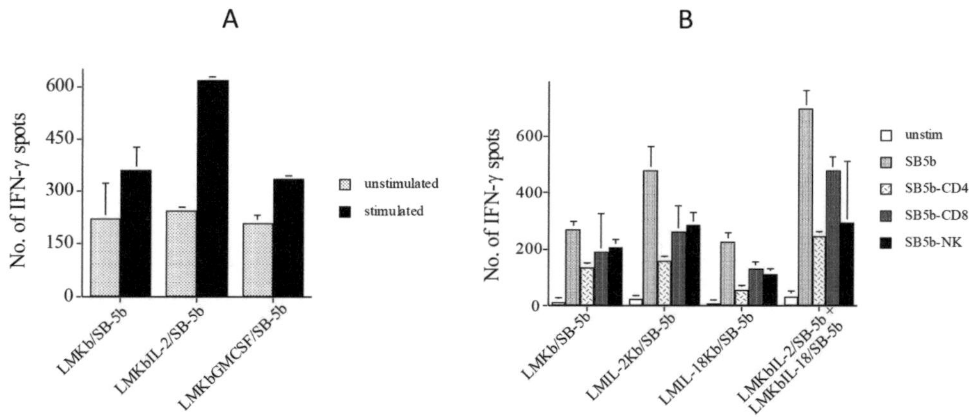

Figure 5.
The proportion of T-cells responsive to tumor cells in mice bearing an i.c. tumor immunized i.c. with DNA-transfected cells modified to secrete IL-2, GM-CSF or IL-18. ELISPOT assay detecting INF- secretion by spleen cells reactive with SB-5b cells in mice immunized with transfected fibroblasts modified to secrete IL-2 or GM-CSF. These animals survived for six weeks following the initial intracerebral injection of SB-5b tumor. The results indicated that the highest proportion of T-cells from the spleens reactive with SB-5b cells were in surviving mice injected with fibroblasts modified to secrete IL-2. Lesser numbers of spots were found in T-cells from mice injected with SB-5b cells and non-secreting transfected fibroblasts or SB-5b cells and transfected fibroblasts modified to secrete GM-CSF. The effect of mAbs against T-cell subsets or NK/LAK cells on the anti-tumor cytotoxic activities of spleen cells from C3H/He mice injected i.c. with a mixture of SB-5b tumor cells and the cytokine-secreting cells transfected with tumor DNA. The animals were injected with a mixture of 1.0 X 10^4 SB-5b tumor cells and 1.0 X 10^6 cytokine-secreting fibroblasts transfected with tumor DNA. Two weeks after the injection, mononuclear cells from the spleens of the immunized mice were used for the ELISPOT assay detecting INF- producing cells. The overall P-value between unstimulated vs. tumor cell stimulated group is $P < 0.001$. The error bars represent one standard deviation.

2.7 Importance of various treatment cells in the development of the antitumor immune response

To analyze the development of systemic anti-tumor immunity in tumor-free mice injected i.c. with cells from the various treatment groups, ELISPOT IFN- assays for measurement of responding T-cells were done using cells from the cervical lymph nodes and spleens from the injected mice. A micro cannula was placed into the right frontal lobe of naive C3H/He mice. Following the cannula insertion, the animals were injected into the brain through the cannula with 1.0 X 10^6 cells from the immuno^{high} pool on 2 days separated by 1 week. As controls, the same procedure was followed except that the cells from the non-enriched master pool or cells from the immuno^{low} pool were substituted for cells from the immuno^{high} pool. As additional controls, the tumor-bearing mice were injected into the brain with equivalent numbers of non-DNA-transfected LMK^b cells or the mice were injected with SB5b tumor cells alone. Mice injected with SB5b tumor cells received only one injection. The data revealed that the highest number of responding T-cells were in the cervical lymph nodes (6A) or spleens (6B) of mice injected i.c. with cells from the immuno^{high} pool ($P < 0.05$) (**Figure 6**).

2.8 Stimulation of T-cell subsets in the spleens of mice with i.c. breast cancer following treatment of the tumor with cells from the immunohigh pool

The number of responding T-cells in the spleens of mice with i.c. breast cancer treated with Cytokine-secreting cells from the various treatment groups was

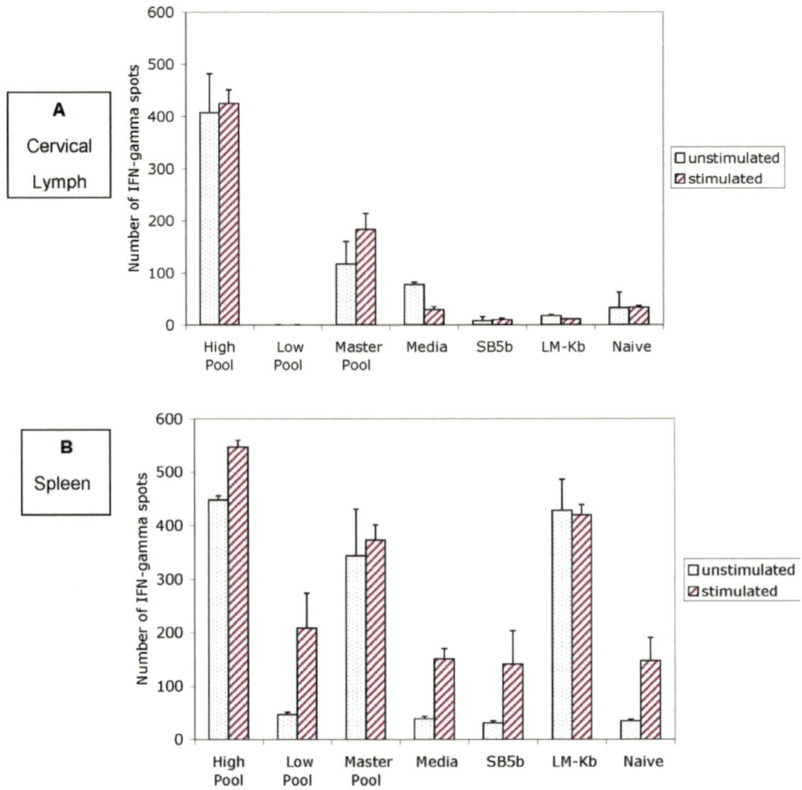

Figure 6.
Increased numbers of responding T-cells were detected in the spleens and cervical lymph nodes of naïve mice which were injected i.c. with cells from the various treatment groups. To determine if systemic anti-tumor immunity was generated in tumor-free mice injected i.c. with cells from the immuno^{high} pool, cervical lymph node and spleen cells from the injected mice were analyzed by ELISPOT IFN- assays for responding T-cells. Naïve C3H/He mice received 2 i.c. injections at weekly intervals of 1.0 X 10^6 cells from the immuno^{high} pool. One week after the second injection, mononuclear cells from the spleens and cervical lymph nodes of the immunized mice were analyzed for the presence of T-cells responsive to the breast cancer cells. As controls, an equivalent number of cells from the non-selected master pool or cells from the immuno^{low} pool were substituted for cells from the immuno^{high} pool. As additional controls, the same protocol was followed except that the mice were injected i.c. with equivalent numbers of SB5b cells, with LMK^b cells or with media. Mice injected with SB5b tumor cells received only one injection. The results illustrated in this figure indicate that the highest number of responding cervical lymph nodes (A) or spleen cells (B) were in mice injected i.c. with cells from the immuno^{high} pool ($p < 0.05$ versus the number of responding spleen cells in mice injected with cells from the master pool and $p < 0.005$ vs. cells from mice in any of the other groups from the cervical lymph nodes).

determined using ELISPOT IFN- assays. A micro cannula was placed into the right frontal lobe of C3H/He mice, and SB5b cells (1.0 X 10^5 in 30 µl) were introduced into the brain through the cannula. On days 2 and 9 following the introduction of tumor, the animals were injected through the cannula into the tumor bed with cells from the immuno^{high} pool. The results (**Figure** 7) reveal that the strongest anti-tumor immune response developed in the spleens of mice with i.c. breast cancer treated i.c. with cells from the immuno^{high} pool ($p < 0.05$) versus the number of responding spleen cells treated with the master pool or any of the other groups.

The effect of antibodies against various T-cell subsets on the responding T-cell response was used to determine the types of cells activated for antitumor immunity in the spleens of mice treated with cells from the immuno^{high} pool using the protocol described above. ELISPOT IFN- assays were used for this analysis. The antitumor

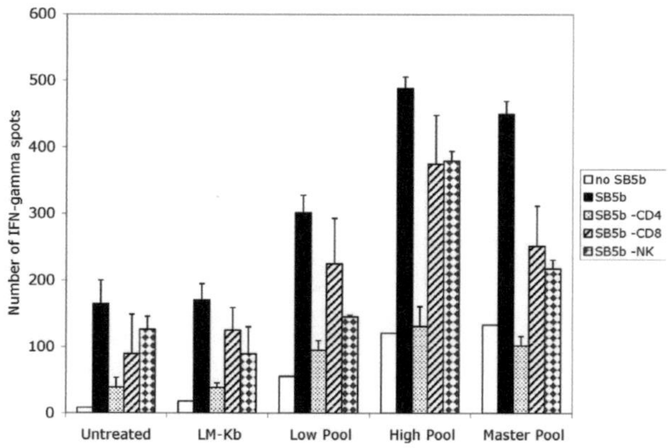

Figure 7.
The effect of antibodies against various T-cell subsets on the cytotoxic response in mice with i.c. breast cancer treated with cells of the various treatment groups. A cannula was placed into the right frontal lobe of C3H/He mice. One day later, the animals received an i.c. injection through the cannula of 1.0 X 10^4 SB5b breast carcinoma cells. On days 2 and 9 following the introduction of tumor, the animals were injected through the cannula into the tumor bed with 1.0 X 10^6 cells from the immuno^{high} pool of transfected cells. As controls, the same procedure was followed except for equivalent numbers of cells from the immuno^{low} pool, the non-selected master pool or non-transfected LMK^b cells were substituted for cells from the immuno^{high} pool. Two weeks after the injection of tumor cells, mononuclear cells from the spleens of the mice were co-incubated with (stimulated) or without (un-stimulated) SB5b cells. The ratio of spleen cells: SB5b cells = 10:1, and the number of INF- spots/10^6 spleen cells is measured. Reduced numbers of spots were detected in spleen cells from mice with i.c. breast cancer injected with cells from the immuno^{high} pool ($p < 0.025$), master pool ($p < 0.025$) or immuno^{low} pool ($p < 0.05$) co-incubated with mAbs for CD4 cells versus the number of spots in the absence of mAbs for CD4 cells.

immune response was inhibited to the greatest extent by antibodies against CD4$^+$ cells (**Figure 7**). The results were less dramatic if the spleen cells were incubated in the media containing CD8$^+$ or NK/LAK antibodies.

2.9 Decreased number of T-reg cells in the spleens of mice with i.c. breast cancer treated with cells from the immunohigh pool

Potent inhibition of antitumor immunity is regulated by T-reg cells [67]. The success of immunotherapeutic protocols depends in part upon the relative numbers of T-reg cells and cytotoxic T lymphocytes in tumor-bearing animals and patients. Quantitative RT-PCR for Foxp3, a transcription factor characteristic of T-reg cells, was used to estimate the relative proportions of T-reg cells in the spleens and brains of mice with i.c. breast cancer injected into the tumor bed with cells from the immuno^{high} pool of transfected cells. Naïve C3H/He mice were injected i.c. with 5.0 X 10^4 SB5b cells along with 1.0 X 10^6 cells from the immuno^{high} pool of transfected cells. The animals received a second i.c. injection of cells from the immuno^{high} pool through the same burr hole. As controls, the same procedure was followed except that the mice were injected with equivalent numbers of SB5b cells and cells from the non-enriched master pool or the immuno^{low} pool. The results (**Figure 8A,B**) indicate that Foxp3$^+$ T-reg cells were relatively deficient in the spleens but not in the brains of animals injected with cells from the immuno^{high} pool. An analysis by FACS of spleen cells from mice injected i.c. with cells from the immuno^{high} pool also revealed a relative deficiency of CD4$^+$/CD25$^+$/Foxp3$^+$ T-cells and a corresponding increase in the relative numbers of CD8$^+$ cells in the spleen (**Figure 8C**) from these animals.

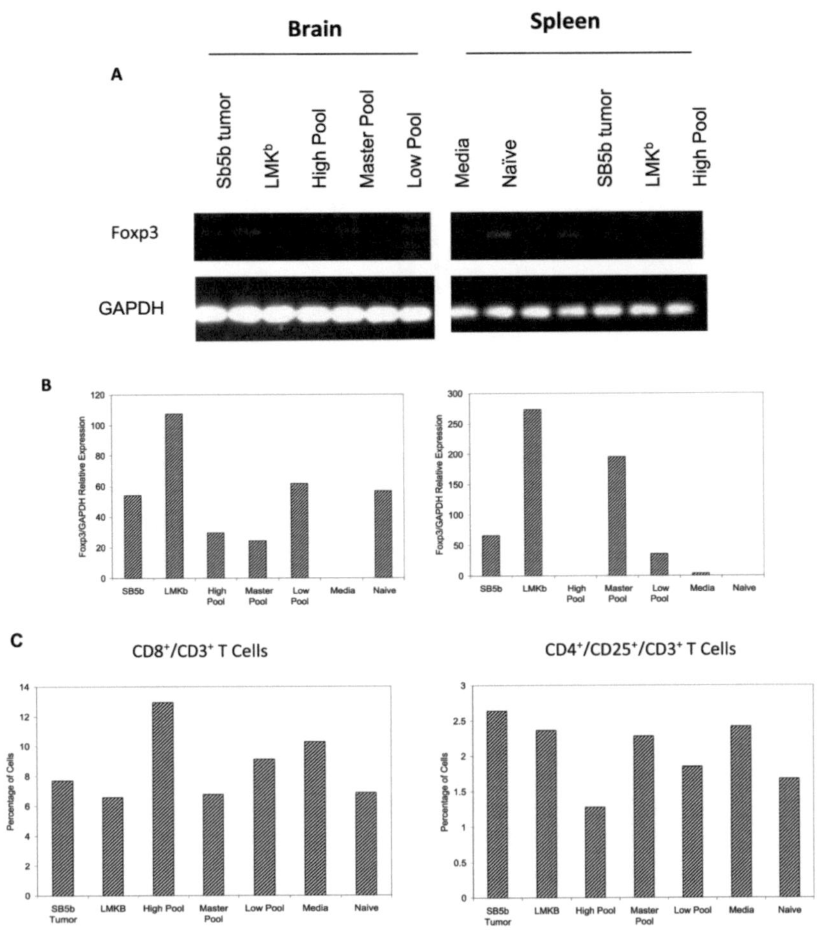

Figure 8.
T-reg cells in the spleens of mice injected with i.c. breast cancer and allogeneic fibroblasts from the various treatment groups. RT-PCR for Foxp3 in the brains and spleens of mice injected i.c. with a mixture of breast cancer cells and cells from the immuno^{high} pool of transfected cells. C3H/He mice received an injection of 5.0 X 10^4 SB5b cells and 1.0 X 10^6 cells from the immuno^{high} pool of transfected cells through a small burr hole. One week later the animals received a second injection of cells from the immuno^{high} pool through the same small burr hole. As controls, the same protocol was followed except that the mice were injected with equivalent numbers of SB5b cells along with cells from the immuno^{low} pool, the non-selected master pool, non-transfected LMK^b cells or the mice were injected with SB5b cells alone. The animals that received SB5b tumor cells were given only one injection. One week after the last injection, mononuclear cells from the tumor bed and the spleen were analyzed by RT-PCR for the expression of Foxp3. Expression of Foxp3 by cells from the tumor bed. The intensity of the amplified 400 bp Foxp3 band, relative to that of the internal control, GAPDH. An analysis by FACS of the spleens of the injected animals shown below revealed a relative deficiency of CD4$^+$/CD25$^+$/Foxp3$^+$ T-reg T-cells and a corresponding increase in the relative numbers of CD8$^+$ cells in the spleens of mice injected i.c. with cells from the immuno^{high} pool. Two weeks following the first injection of tumor and treatment cells, mononuclear cells from the spleens of three immunized mice were harvested and pooled for analysis by FACS. Each of the following steps was performed on ice. Tissues were minced and finely homogenized using a razor blade in 5 ml of serum-free DMEM. The homogenate was spun down and re-suspended in fresh, ice-cold serum-free DMEM. Single-cell suspension was obtained by filtration through 70-μm nylon mesh into sterile 50-ml conical tubes. The cells were centrifuged to form a pellet and the supernatant was poured off. The supernatant was subsequently removed and the cell pellet was re-suspended in ACK lysis buffer for 5 minutes, and spun down. The pellet was washed in 5 ml of PSS and spun down. All pellets were re-suspended in 5 ml of FACS buffer (5% bovine serum albumin and 5% heat-inactivated horse serum), incubated (4°C) for 5 min, spun down to a pellet and resuspended in 5 ml of PBS. Data is expressed as a percentage of gated cells from the entire population of spleen cells.

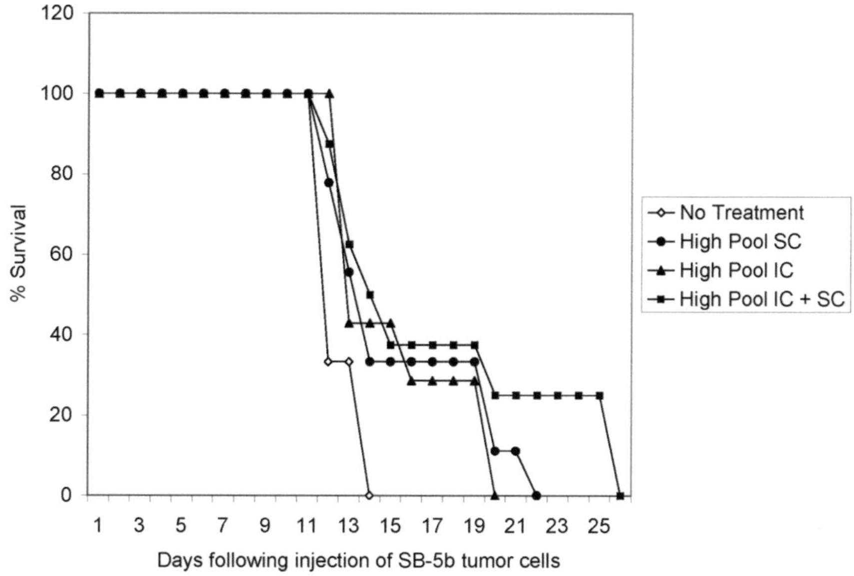

Figure 9.
Survival of mice with i.c. breast cancer treated by immunization with cells from the immuno^{high} pool of transfected cells. C3H/He mice (eight animals/group) were injected with 5.0 X 10^4 SB5b cells and 1.0 X 10^6 cells from the immuno^{high} pool through a small burr hole. At the same time animals with i.c. tumor were injected s.c. (subcutaneously) with an equivalent number of cells from the immuno^{high} pool alone or both i.c. and s.c. with cells from the immuno^{high} pool. Mean survival time (MST) in days: Injected with SB5b alone, 12.7 ± 1.0; injected with SB5b and cells from immuno^{high} pool s.c., 15.6 ± 3.9; injected with SB5b cells and cells from immuno^{high} pool i.c., 15.4 ± 3.3; injected with SB5b cells and cells from the immuno^{high} pool i.c. and s.c., 17.4 ± 5.9. Probability values were as follows: $p < 0.05$ for mice injected with SB5b cells and cells from the immuno^{high} pool s.c., i.c. or i.c. and s.c. versus untreated mice.

3. Prolonged survival of mice with i.c. breast cancer upon treatment by injection into the tumor bed with cells from the immunohigh pool

To explore the potential prolongation of survival in mice with i.c. breast cancer treated by cells from the immuno^{high} pool, C3H/He mice were injected i.c. with 5.0 X 10^4 SB5b cells and 1.0 X 10^6 cells from the immuno^{high} pool. The findings from these studies (**Figure 9**) revealed that mice with i.c. breast cancer treated with cells from the immuno^{high} pool survived significantly longer than untreated mice ($p < 0.05$). Similar results were demonstrated if the mice with i.c. breast cancer cells were treated with subcutaneous (s.c.) injection of cells from the immuno^{high} pool.

4. Conclusions

Patients with primary or metastatic tumors in the brain continue to experience a limited survival which has not improved over many years. There is an urgent need for new and more effective forms of treatment for these patients. Immunotherapy, which is designed to stimulate an antitumor immune response to various tumors is beginning to show potential for several different types of cancer. Cytokine expression in tumors is a strategy to stimulate potent activation of the immune system. The use of cytokines has become more common in the treatment of patients with high-grade gliomas, particularly with IL-2 and IL-15 [68, 69]. A potential advantage of IL-15 is that there is less activation of immune inhibitory Tregs associated with this cytokine [19]. Preliminary results, however, have not demonstrated a robust efficacy for prolonging survival in patients with brain tumors using various cytokines including IL-2 or IL-15 [70].

In the studies presented here, a significant prolongation of survival was observed with two different oncolytic poxviruses expressing the IL15Rα-IL15 fusion protein in combination with a prostaglandin synthesis inhibitor to block immunosuppression. Oncolytic viruses may contribute to the anti-tumor response by a direct cytotoxic effect on cancer cells associated with the release of tumor antigens that may stimulate an immune response. Previous studies have shown that the oncolytic poxvirus, myxoma virus, is safe to use in mice even when directly injected into the cerebral ventricles.

When the virus is engineered to express a cytokine such as IL-15, it can stimulate local expression of potent immune-activating agents, while avoiding systemic inflammation that parenteral delivery of the cytokine would produce. In this study, IL15 was chosen because it activates and maintains the function of NK and $CD8^+$ T-cells [71] with less vascular leakage potential [72] and less activation of Tregs.

In addition, there is less activation-induced cell death for $CD8^+$ effector T-cells with this cytokine. In summary, the data suggests that a poxvirus genetically engineered to secrete IL-15 along with an anti-immuno-suppressant is an effective treatment strategy in prolonging survival in mice with a malignant glioma.

In other studies, it was shown that the enhanced immunotherapeutic properties of a vaccine prepared by transfer of a cDNA expression library derived from tumor cells into a mouse fibroblast cell line engineered to secrete IL-2 also appears to have significant potential in the treatment of a brain tumor. The cDNA integrates spontaneously into the genome of the recipient cells followed by replication and expression. The vaccine can be prepared from small amounts of tumor tissue, enabling treatment at an early stage of the disease, when tumor tissue is available in only limited amounts and the tumor is most susceptible to immune-based therapy. A unique enrichment strategy has also been developed such that the proportion of active immunotherapeutic cells in the vaccine is increased.

The use of cells from the enriched vaccine was associated with the development of a strong antitumor immune response. Cells from the ($immuno^{high}$) pool were injected into the tumor bed of mice with intracerebral breast cancer, and this resulted in a prolongation of survival in the treated mice. ELISPOT IFN-γ assays revealed significantly elevated anti-tumor immune responses in spleen cell populations derived from tumor-bearing mice injected i.c. with cells from the $immuno^{high}$ pools. The injection of cells from various control groups including cells from the $immuno^{low}$ pools did not reveal significant anti-tumor immune responses. The predominant cell type activated in mice immunized with cells from the the $immuno^{high}$ pool were $CD4^+$ T-cells. Injection of cells from the $immuno^{high}$ pool into the tumor bed also resulted in a reduction of the relative numbers of T-reg cells with a potential prevention of the impaired anti-tumor immune responses frequently found in patients with malignant brain tumors.

The goal of tumor treatment would be the removal of every tumor cell. It is unlikely that a single therapy can achieve this goal in the case of brain tumors. However, immunotherapy in combination with surgical removal of the tumor, radiation therapy and chemotherapy will likely be involved in the treatment of patients with brain tumors. The development of DNA-based tumor vaccines in combination with cytokine secretion is a novel strategy that does not require antigen identification or protein purification and yet can elicit a potent and long-lasting activation of the immune response, which will lead to the rejection of the tumor. From a practical point of view, these vaccines are easy to prepare, and they are relatively inexpensive. Only small quantities of tumor-derived DNA are needed, which can be obtained from small surgical specimens. The enrichment strategy represents a unique approach to isolating highly immunogenic pools of transfected cells which leads to the development of enhanced anti-tumor immunity. Thus DNA-based cytokine-secreting vaccines offer several unique advantages, which support their further development for cancer immunotherapy in general and specifically for the treatment of patients with malignant intracerebral tumors. The use of viruses engineered to secrete cytokines remains another treatment option for further study regarding the management of these tumors.

Author details

Terry Lichtor[1*], Bingtao Tang[2] and Edward J. Roy[2]

1 Department of Neurological Surgery, Rush University Medical Center, Chicago, Illinois, USA

2 Department of Molecular and Integrative Physiology, University of Illinois at Urbana-Champaign, Urbana, IL, USA

*Address all correspondence to: terry_lichtor@rush.edu

References

[1] Ries LAG, Kosary CL, Hankey BF, Miller BA, Edwards BK. SEER Cancer Statistics Review, 1973-1995. Bethesda, MD: National Cancer Institute; 1988

[2] Imperato JP, Paleologos NA, Vick NA. Effects of treatment on long-term survivors with malignant atrocytomas. Annals of Neurology. 1990;**28**:818-822

[3] Heimans JJ, Taphoorn MJ. Impact of brain tumor treatment on quality of life. Journal of Neurology. 2002;**249**:955-960

[4] Belanich M, Randall T, Pastor MA, Kibitel JT, Alas LG, Dolan ME, et al. Intracellular localization and intercellular heterogeneity of the human DNA repair protein O(6)-methylguanine-DNA methyltransferase. Cancer Chemotherapy and Pharmacology. 1996;**37**:547-555

[5] Hotta T, Saito Y, Fujita H, Mikami T, Kurisu K, Kiya K, et al. O6-alkylguanine-DNA alkyltransferase activity of human malignant glioma and its clinical implications. Journal of Neuro-Oncology. 1994;**21**:135-140

[6] Insug O, Ku G, Ertl HCJ, Blaszczyk-Thurin M. A dendritic cell vaccine induces protective immunity to intracranial growth of glioma. Anticancer Research. 2002;**22**:613-622

[7] Rosenberg SA, Yang JC, Restifo NP. Cancer immunotherapy: Moving beyond current vaccines. Nature Medicine. 2004;**10**:909-915

[8] Kobayashi T, Yamanaka R, Homma J, Tsuchiya N, Yajima N, Yoshida S, et al. Tumor mRNA-loaded dendritic cells elicit tumor-specific $CD8^+$ cytotoxic T cells in patients with malignant glioma. Cancer Immunology, Immunotherapy. 2003;**52**:632-637

[9] Finocchiaro G, Pellegatta S. Immunotherapy with dendritic cells loaded with glioblastoma stem cells: From preclinical to clinical studies. Cancer Immunology and Immunotherapy. 2016;**65**:101-109

[10] Reardon DA, Gilbert MR, Wick W, Liau L. Immunotherapy for neuro-oncology: The critical rationale for combinatorial therapy. Neuro Oncology. 2015;**17**(Suppl. 7):vii32-vii40

[11] Lichtor T, Glick RP, Feldman LA, OsawaG,HardmanJ,O-SullivanI,CohenEP. Enhanced immunity to intracerebral breast cancer in mice immunized with a cDNA-based vaccine enriched for immunotherapeutic cells. Journal of Immunotherapy. 2008;**31**:18-27

[12] Chang AL, Miska J, Wainwright DA, Dey M, Rivetta CV, Yu D, et al. CCL2 produced by the glioma microenvironment is essential for the recruitment of regulatory T cells and myeloid-derived suppressor cells. Cancer Research. 2016;**76**:5671-5682

[13] Ooi YC, Tran P, Ung N, Thill K, Trang A, Fong BM, et al. The role of regulatory T-cells in glioma immunology. Clinical Neurology and Neurosurgery. 2014;**119**:125-132

[14] Lan Y, Zhang D, Xu C, Hance KW, Marelli B, Qi J, et al. Enhanced preclinical antitumor activity of M7824, a bifunctional fusion protein simultaneously targeting PD-Li and TGF-β. Science Translational Medicine. 2018;**10**(424):eaan5488. DOI: 10-1126/scitranlmed.aan5488

[15] Mostofa AGM, Punganuru SR, Madala HR, Al-Obaide M, Srivenugopal KS. The process and

regulatory components of inflammation in brain oncogenesis. Biomolecules. 2017;7(2):34. DOI: 10.3390/biom7020034

[16] Steel JC, Waldmann A, Morris JC. Interleukin-15 biology and its therapeutic implications in cancer. Trends in Permacology Sciences. 2012;**33**:35-41

[17] Wrangle JM, Patterson A, Johnson CB, Neitzke DJ, Mehrotra S, Denlinger CE, et al. IL-2 and beyond in cancer immunotherapy. Journal of Interferon & Cytokine Research. 2018;**38**:45-68

[18] Cheever MA. Twelve immunotherapy drugs that could cure cancers. Immunological Reviews. 2008;**222**:357-368

[19] Berger C, Berger M, Hackman RC, Gough M, Elliott C, Jensen MC, et al. Safety and immunologic effects of IL-15 administration in nonhuman primates. Blood. 2009;**114**:2417-2426

[20] Gansbacher B, Bannerji R, Daniels B, Zier K, Cronin K, Gilboa E. Retroviral vector-mediated gamma-interferon gene transfer into tumor cells generates potent and long-lasting antitumor immunity. Cancer Research. 1990;**50**:7820-7825

[21] Colombo MP, Ferrari G, Stoppacciaro A, Parenza M, Rodolfo M, Mavilio F, et al. Granulocyte colony-stimulating factor gene transfer suppressed tumorigenicity of a murine adenocarcinoma *in vivo*. The Journal of Experimental Medicine. 1991;**173**:889-897

[22] Golumbek PT, Lazenby AJ, Levitsky HI, Jaffee LM, Karasuyama H, Baker M, et al. Treatment of established renal cancer by tumor cells engineered to secrete interleukin-4. Science. 1991;**254**:713-716

[23] Mullen CA, Coale MM, Levy AT, Stetler-Stevenson WG, Liotta LA, Brandt S, et al. Fibrosarcoma cells transduced with the IL-6 gene exhibit reduced tumorigenicity, increased immunogenicity, and decreased metastatic potential. Cancer Research. 1992;**52**:6020-6024

[24] Dranoff G, Jaffee E, Lazenby A, Golumbek P, Levitsky H, Brose K, et al. Vaccination with irradiated tumor cells engineered to secrete murine granulocyte-macrophage colony-stimulating factor stimulates potent, specific and long-lasting anti-tumor immunity. Proceedings of the National Academy of Sciences of the United States of America. 1993;**90**:3539-3543

[25] Connor J, Bannerji R, Saito S, Heston W, Fair W, Gilboa E. Regression of bladder tumors in mice treated with interleukin 2 gene-modified tumor cells. The Journal of Experimental Medicine. 1993;**177**:1127-1111

[26] Cavallo F, Pierro FD, Giovarelli M, Gulino A, Vacca A, Stoppacciaro A, et al. Protective and curative potential of vaccination with interleukin-2-gene-transfected cells from a spontaneous mouse mammary adenocarcinoma. Cancer Research. 1993;**53**:5067-5070

[27] Tahara H, Zeh HJ, Storkus WJ, Pappo I, Watkins SC, Gubler U, et al. Fibroblasts genetically engineered to secrete interleukin 12 can suppress tumor growth and induce antitumor immunity to a murine melanoma *in vivo*. Cancer Research. 1994;**54**:182-189

[28] Yu JS, Wei MX, Chiocca EA, Martuza RL, Tepper RI. Treatment of glioma by engineered interleukin 4-secreting cells. Cancer Research. 1993;**53**:3125-3128

[29] Bommareddy PK, Shettigar M, Kaufman HL. Integrating oncolytic viruses in combination cancer immunotherapy. Nature Reviews. Immunology. 2018;**18**:498-513

[30] Jayawardena N, Poirier JT, Burga LN, Bostina M. Virus-receptor interactions and virus neutralization: Insights for oncolytic virus development. Oncolytic Virotherapy. 2020;**9**:1-15

[31] Wang G, Barrett JW, Stanford M, Werden SJ, Johnston JB, Gao X, et al. Infection of human cancer cells with myxoma virus requires Akt activation via interaction with a viral ankyrin-repeat host range factor. Proceedings of the National Academy of Sciences. 2006;**103**:4640-4645

[32] Werden SJ, McFadden G. The role of cell signaling in poxvirus tropism: The case of the M-T5 host range protein of myxoma virus. Biochimica et Biophysica Acta (BBA) - Proteins and Proteomics. 2008;**1784**:228-237

[33] Parato KA, Breitbach CJ, Le Boeuf F, Wang J, Storbeck C, Ilkow C, et al. The oncolytic poxvirus JX-594 selectively replicates in and destroys cancer cells driven by genetic pathways commonly activated in cancers. Molecular Therapy. 2012;**20**:749-758

[34] Bartee E, Mohamed MR, Lopez MC, Baker HV, McFadden G. The addition of tumor necrosis factor plus Beta interferon induces a novel synergistic antiviral state against poxviruses in primary human fibroblasts. Journal of Virology. 2009;**83**:498-511

[35] Bartee E, McFadden G. Human cancer cells have specifically lost the ability to induce the synergistic state caused by tumor necrosis factor plus interferon-beta. Cytokine. 2009;**47**:199-205

[36] Kim M, Williamson CT, Prudhomme J, Bebb DG, Riabowol K, Lee PWK, et al. The viral tropism of two distinct oncolytic viruses, reovirus and myxoma virus, is modulated by cellular tumor suppressor gene status. Oncogene. 2010;**29**:3990-3996

[37] Rahman MM, McFadden G. Oncolytic virotherapy with myxoma virus. Journal of Clinical Medicine. 2020;**9**:171. DOI: 10.3390/jcm9010171

[38] Guo ZS, Lu B, Guo Z, Giehl E, Feist M, Dai E, et al. Vaccinia virus-mediated cancer immunotherapy: Cancer vaccines and oncolytics. Journal for Immunotherapy of Cancer. 2019;7(1):6. DOI: 10.1186/s40425-018-0495-7

[39] Johnson DB, Puzanov I, Kelley MC. Talimogene laherparepvec (T-VEC) for the treatment of advanced melanoma. Immunotherapy. 2015;7:611-619

[40] Bommareddy PK, Patel A, Hossain S, Kaufman HL. Talimogene laherparepvec (T-VEC) and other oncolytic viruses for the treatment of melanoma. American Journal of Clinical Dermatology. 2017;**18**:1-15

[41] Liu BL, Robinson M, Han ZQ, Branston RH, English C, Reay P, et al. ICP34.5 deleted herpes simplex virus with enhanced oncolytic, immune stimulating, and anti-tumour properties. Gene Therapy. 2003;**10**:292-303

[42] Franke V, Berger DMS, Klop WMC, van der Hiel B, van de Wiel BA, Ter Meulen S, et al. High response rates for T-VEC in early metastatic melanoma (stage IIIB/C-IVM1a). International Journal of Cancer. 2019;**145**:974-978

[43] Kelly CM, Antonescu CR, Bowler T, Munhoz R, Chi P, Dickson MA, et al. Objective response rate among patients with locally advanced or metastatic sarcoma treated with talimogene laherparepvec in combination with pembrolizumab: A phase 2 clinical trial. JAMA Oncology. 2020;**6**:402-408

[44] Todo T, Martuza RL, Rabkin SD, Johnson PA. Oncolytic herpes simplex virus vector with enhanced MHC class

I presentation and tumor cell killing. Proceedings of the National Academy of Sciences. 2001;**98**:6396-6401

[45] Todo T, ATIM-14. Results of phase II clinical trial of oncolytic herpes virus G47Δ in patients with glioblastoma. Neuro-Oncology. 2019;**21**(Issue Supplement):vi4

[46] Gromeier M, Alexander L, Wimmer E. Internal ribosomal entry site substitution eliminates neurovirulence in intergeneric poliovirus recombinants. Proceedings of the National Academy of Sciences. 1996;**93**:2370-2375

[47] Desjardins A, Gromeier M, Herndon JE 2nd, Beaubier N, Bolognesi DP, Friedman AH, et al. Recurrent glioblastoma treated with recombinant poliovirus. The New England Journal of Medicine. 2018;**379**:150-161

[48] Holl EK, Brown MC, Boczkowski D, McNamara MA, George DJ, Bigner DD, et al. Recombinant oncolytic poliovirus, PVSRIPO, has potent cytotoxic and innate inflammatory effects, mediating therapy in human breast and prostate cancer xenograft models. Oncotarget. 2016;**7**:79828-79841

[49] Toyoda H, Yin J, Mueller S, Wimmer E, Cello J. Oncolytic treatment and cure of neuroblastoma by a novel attenuated poliovirus in a novel poliovirus-susceptible animal model. Cancer Research. 2007;**67**:2857-2864

[50] Fields BN, Knipe DM, Howley PM. Fields Virology. Philadelphia, PA, USA: Wolters Kluwer Health/Lippincott Williams & Wilkins; 2013

[51] Smith GL, Moss B. Infectious poxvirus vectors have capacity for at least 25 000 base pairs of foreign DNA. Gene. 1983;**25**:21-28

[52] Kowalsky SJ, Liu Z, Feist M, Berkey SE, Ma C, Ravindranathan R, et al. Superagonist IL-15-armed oncolytic virus elicits potent antitumor immunity and therapy that are enhanced by PD-1 blockade. Molecular Therapy. 2018;**26**:2476-2486

[53] Tang B, Guo ZS, Bartlett DL, Yan DZ, Schane CP, Thomas DL, et al. Synergistic combination of oncolytic virotherapy and immunotherapy for glioma. Clinical Cancer Research. 2020;**26**:2216-2230

[54] Zeh HJ, Downs-Canner S, McCart JA, Guo ZS, Rao UN, Ramalingam L, et al. First-in-man study of Western reserve strain oncolytic vaccinia virus: Safety, systemic spread, and antitumor activity. Molecular Therapy. 2015;**23**:202-214

[55] Downs-Canner S, Guo ZS, Ravindranathan R, Breitbach CJ, O'Malley ME, Jones HL, et al. Phase 1 study of intravenous oncolytic poxvirus (vvDD) in patients with advanced solid cancers. Molecular Therapy. 2016;**24**:1492-1501

[56] Tang B, Guo ZS, Bartlett DL, Liu J, McFadden G, Shisler JL, et al. A cautionary note on the selectivity of oncolytic poxviruses. Oncolytic Virotherapy. 2019;**8**:3-8

[57] Niemann J, Woller N, Brooks J, Fleischmann-Mundt B, Martin NT, Kloos A, et al. Molecular retargeting of antibodies converts immune defense against oncolytic viruses into cancer immunotherapy. Nature Communications. 2019;**10**:3236

[58] Fulci G, Dmitrieva N, Gianni D, Fontana EJ, Pan X, Lu Y, et al. Depletion of peripheral macrophages and brain microglia increases brain tumor titers of oncolytic viruses. Cancer Research. 2007;**67**:9398-9406

[59] Alvarez-Breckenridge CA, Yu J, Price R, Wojton J, Pradarelli J, Mao H, et al. NK cells impede glioblastoma virotherapy through NKp30 and NKp46 natural cytotoxicity receptors. Nature Medicine. 2012;**18**:1827-1834

[60] Lichtor T, Glick RP, Kim TS, Hand R, Cohen EP. Prolonged survival of mice with glioma injected intracerebrally with double cytokine-secreting cells. Journal of Neurosurgery. 1995;**83**:1038-1044

[61] Lun XQ, Jang J-H, Tang N, Deng H, Head R, Bell JC, et al. Efficacy of systemically administered oncolytic vaccinia virotherapy for malignant gliomas is enhanced by combination therapy with rapamycin or cyclophosphamide. Clinical Cancer Research. 2009;**15**:2777-2788

[62] Stanford MM, Barrett JW, Nazarian SH, Werden S, McFadden G. Oncolytic virotherapy synergism with signaling inhibitors: Rapamycin increases myxoma virus tropism for human tumor cells. Journal of Virology. 2007;**81**:1251-1260

[63] Thomas DL, Doty R, Tosic V, Liu J, Kranz DM, McFadden G, et al. Myxoma virus combined with rapamycin treatment enhances adoptive T cell therapy for murine melanoma brain tumors. Cancer Immunology, Immunotherapy. 2011;**60**:1461-1472

[64] Seibert K, Masferrer JL. Role of inducible cyclooxygenase (COX-2) in inflammation. Receptor. 1994;**4**:17-23

[65] Tang B, Foss K, Lichtor T, Phillips H, Roy E. Resection of orthotopic murine brain glioma. Neuroimmunology and Neuroinflammation. 2021;**8**:64-69. DOI: 10.20517/2347-8659.2020.28

[66] Lichtor T, Glick RP, Lin H, Sullivan OI, Cohen EP. Intratumoral injection of IL-secreting syngeneic/allogeneic fibroblasts transfected with DNA from breast cancer cells prolongs the survival of mice with intracerebral breast cancer. Cancer Gene Therapy. 2005;**12**:708-714

[67] Fecci PE, Mitchell DA, Whitesides JF, Xie W, Friedman AH, Archer GE, et al. Increased regulatory T-cell function amidst a diminished CD4 compartment explains cellular immune defects in patients with malignant glioma. Cancer Research. 2006;**66**:3294-3202

[68] Zhenjiang L, Rao M, Luo X, Valentini D, Von Landenberg A, Meng Q, et al. Cytokine networks and surviving peptide-specific cellular immune responses predict improved survival in patients with gliobastoma multiforme. eBioMedicine. 2018;**33**:49-56

[69] Zhan Q, Zhang HJ, Wang Om Zhu G, Jin G, Fusheng L. Glioma-associated mesenchymal stem cells-mediated PD-L1 expression is attenuated by AD5-Ki67-15 in GBM treatment. Stem Cell Research & Therapy. 2022;**13**:284

[70] Medikonda R, Pant A, Lim M. Immunotherapy as a new therapeutic approach for brain and spinal cord tumors. Advances in Experimental Medicine and Biology. 2023;**1394**:73-84

[71] Jakobisiak M, Golab J, Lasek W. Interleukin 15 as a promising candidate for tumor immunotherapy. Cytokine & Growth Factor Reviews. 2011;**22**:99-108

[72] Munger W, DeJoy SQ, Jeyaseelan R, Torley LW, Grabstein KH, Eisenmann J, et al. Studies evaluating the antitumor activity and toxicity of interleukin-15, a new T cell growth factor: Comparison with Interleukin-2. Cellular Immunology. 1995;**165**:289-293

Chapter 2

Attributing Meaning to Molecular Interaction Networks by Leveraging Clinical and Omic Data: The Missing Link between Tumor Biology and Treatment Strategies in Glioma

Andra V. Krauze

Abstract

The pace of data growth in the molecular space has led to the evolution of sophisticated approaches to data aggregation and linkages, such as IPA, STRING, KEGG, and others. These tools aim to generate molecular interaction networks harnessing growing molecular data at all levels to link tumor biology knowledge to signaling pathways and matched analyses. Potentially actionable biomarkers, however, are evaluated based on clinically associated prognosis, and necessary computational approaches should be vetted for interpretability through a clinical lens. Intersectional clinical and computational expertise is needed to link omics, molecular interactions, and clinical data to address the missing link between tumor biology and treatment strategies.

Keywords: molecular interaction networks, omics, tumor biology, biomarkers, clinical

1. Introduction

As increasingly large-scale data streams in genomic, transcriptomic, proteomic, and metabolic contexts are becoming available to researchers, molecular signals are emerging at an unprecedented pace. This rise in data and signal has rightfully fostered the emergence of molecular interaction networks toolsets, including Ingenuity Pathway Analysis (IPA) [1], Search Tool for the Retrieval of Interacting Genes/Proteins (STRING) [2], Kyoto Encyclopedia of Genes and Genomes (KEGG) [3] and others to group, annotate and classify emerging signals. While highly sophisticated and evolving, these interactions directly lead to emerging evidence. Still, they are increasingly more challenging to implement with specified training and expertise, and the pressure for rapid interpretation can render the ongoing generation of information biased and may limit the identification of connections in novel signals.

Despite the rapid rise in signal, the clinical space and clinical implementation functions in a realm driven by studies that generate information wherein one or very few interventions are analyzed with limited molecular data acquired. Often clinical studies are aimed at testing a specific hypothesis but are difficult to link to large-scale data since they carry clinical but relatively less omic data. Clinical links to omic data and molecular interaction networks are lacking, limiting emerging data classification when employing molecular interaction networks. Molecules widely studied reemerge in linkage analyses but still lack a clear mechanistic context that can be effectively exploited for therapeutic gain. Sex differences have increasingly been studied in glioma, but specific classification via molecular interactions is evolving. Equally so, there is no linkage between tumor burden, response to particular interventions over time, and survival endpoints are generally employed with limited data on progression. Some clinical characteristics such as age and sex are linked to prognosis and biological triggers and thus present important avenues for classifying molecular networks to allow for a superior understanding of biology and to identify predictive biomarkers. Signaling routes that are gaining momentum and experience in glioma, including Notch, NF-κB signaling, ferroptosis, the lipidome, fatty acid metabolism, and the propagation, evolution, and sustainment of stem cells, all overlap in interaction and require more research to define in omic terms. Treatment strategies have centered on signals surpassed by rapidly evolving knowledge in the field and do not connect to molecular subtypes emerging in proteogenomic analyses. The emerging rapidly changing landscape of databases and interaction networks is surfacing new connections in large-scale omic data, which will be discussed, highlighting pathways shared among analyses leading into biological mechanisms and therapeutic strategies existing and ongoing to eventually leverage clinical and omic data in glioma.

2. The growing landscape of molecular interaction network databases and connections to glioma

Molecular interaction networks are growing to meet researcher demands, with over 50,000 publications in Web of Science as of mid-2023. Notably, in this context, 21% of publications are related to biochemistry and molecular biology, and 4.3% to oncology. The growth of interest and research in this space is evidenced by a rise in publications from 41 in 2012 to 280 in 2022 [4]. Paralleling this interest in aggregating data into networks is the growth in tools making this possible. There are several reasons for the existence of multiple avenues of aggregating, analyzing, and visualizing molecular data since each meets different needs, either with different data sources or approaches to linkage (**Figure 1**). As toolsets gather information from evidence-based medicine from various sources and aggregate this in classification networks, there is source and data overlap but also distinctions (**Table 1**). STRING (Search Tool for the Retrieval of Interacting Genes/Proteins) gathers protein interaction information from the annotated proteomes maintained by SWISS-PROT with functional information on genes derived from a manually curated orthology database, Clusters of Orthologous Genes (COG) when available and when not available then automatically derived by an automatic method resembling the COG methodology [2] to generate protein association networks. The linkage of data sources that are widely available to other data sources, e.g., TCGA (The Cancer Genome Atlas), CGGA (Chinese Glioma Genome Atlas), and Gene Expression Omnibus (GEO), facilitates the identification of networks and the assignment of meaning to novel protein signals [6]. As exemplified

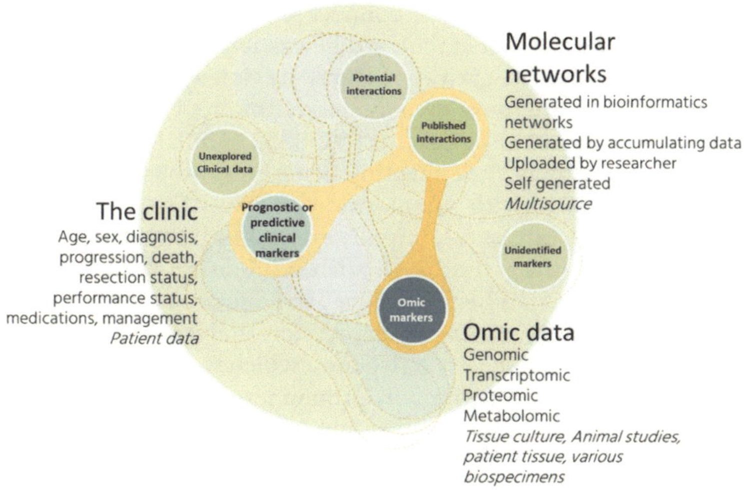

Figure 1.
The complex interplay results in molecular interaction networks based on one-to-one and one-to-many relationships between available clinical data and published omic data. Unexplored clinical data and unidentified or unpublished markers do not connect to molecular networks despite one-to-many relationships between data components [5].

Database	Source of data and output	Usage in literature for Glioma
STRING (Search Tool for the Retrieval of Interacting Genes/ Proteins) [2, 6]	https://string-db.org/ SWISS-PROT, COG Protein-protein interactions	Li et al., 2020 Bioinformatic Profiling of Prognosis-Related Genes in Malignant Glioma Microenvironment [7] Mischkulnig et al. 2022. The impact of heme biosynthesis regulation on glioma aggressiveness: Correlations with diagnostic molecular markers [8]
KEGG (Kyoto Encyclopedia of Genes and Genomes) [3]	https://www.kegg.jp/ Public databases, published literature curation, protein structure databases, genome and chemical databases Pathways, Interactions	Guvem et al., 2022 Screening the Significant Hub Genes by Comparing Tumor Cells, Normoxic, and Hypoxic Glioblastoma Stem-like Cell Lines Using Co-Expression Analysis in Glioblastoma. [9] Li et al., 2022. Identification of a key glioblastoma candidate gene, FUBP3, based on weighted gene co-expression network analysis [10]
IPA (Ingenuity Pathway Analysis) [1]	http://www.ingenuity.com/ Public databases published literature curation, proprietary databases, and researcher-uploaded experimental data Pathways, Interactions	Ghosh et al., 2017. Core Canonical Pathways Involved in Developing Human Glioblastoma Multiforme (GBM) [11] Tasci et al. 2023. RadWise: A Rank-Based Hybrid Feature Weighting and Selection Method for Proteomic Categorization of Chemoirradiation in Patients with Glioblastoma. [12]
WGCNA (Weighted Gene Co-expression Network Analysis) [13]	Data analysis technique Correlated genes and proteins along modules of co-expressed genes	Yang et al. 2018. Candidate Biomarkers and Molecular Mechanism Investigation for Glioblastoma Multiforme Utilizing WGCNA [14] Zhou et al., 2021. Construction of co-expression modules related to survival by WGCNA and identification of potential prognostic biomarkers in glioblastoma. [15]
GSEA (Gene Set Enrichment Analysis) [16]	Gene sets defined based on differential expression Ranked lists of gene sets	Lin et al., 2020. Characterization of Hypoxia Signature to Evaluate the Tumor Immune Microenvironment and Predict Prognosis in Glioma Groups [17]

Table 1.
Major omic interaction databases and bioinformatics applications and connections to glioma literature.

by Li et al., STRING can be employed to connect prognosis-related genes to the glioma microenvironment, which in their study was accomplished by employing TCGA and GSE4290 data sets to arrive at several previously lesser known or unknown genes that share both a link to the glioma microenvironment and prognosis [7]. Mischkulnig et al. employed TCGA data and STRING to link heme biosynthesis regulation to glioma aggressiveness by connecting heme biosynthesis RNA expression to molecular markers associated with glioma grade [8]. The KEGG (Kyoto Encyclopedia of Genes and Genomes) database [3], initially created in 1995, is a conglomerate of 16 databases and functions by gathering published literature to map omic signals to pathways (**Figure 2**). KEGG has been employed to compare normoxic and hypoxic glioblastoma stem-like cell lines using co-expression analysis and linkage to the gene expression dataset GSE117 to identify hub genes, which were then subsequently screened with STRING to examine protein-protein interactions [9]. As an example of linkage of a novel signal, KEGG has been employed to analyze the possible function of FUBP3, identified by Li et al. as the only gene associated with survival out of 5 intersection genes in 2 GEO datasets [10]. FUBP3 was found to have an immunohistochemical expression in GBM and adjacent tissue with KEGG, linking it to association with immune surveillance in GBM. IPA (Ingenuity pathway analysis), developed by Qiagen, is a combination of functional analysis and databases that employs a variety of data sources, including public data and proprietary data, and allows linkage with experimental data uploaded by users of the platform. It also employs manual curation of existing published data to allow for annotation. IPA can thus evolve to include a wide array of canonical pathways, as exemplified by Ghosh et al., with core canonical pathways identified in GBM [11]. As novel omic signals are identified in response to management, these can be linked to canonical pathways [12]. WGCNA (Weighted Gene Co-expression Network Analysis) analyzes proteogenomic connections by generating mapping co-expression of molecules to modules [13]. Candidate biomarkers can thus be linked to molecular mechanisms as exemplified by Yang et al., wherein WGCNA was utilized to link the gene expression profile of GSE50161 to 47 tissue samples, of which 34 were surgical brain tissue samples, 47 from patients with GBM and 13 from normal brain, in this case, pediatric epilepsy patients [14]. In this analysis, the modules identified using WGCNA were examined using an independent TCGA data set to arrive at several molecules that may be utilized as signals in liquid

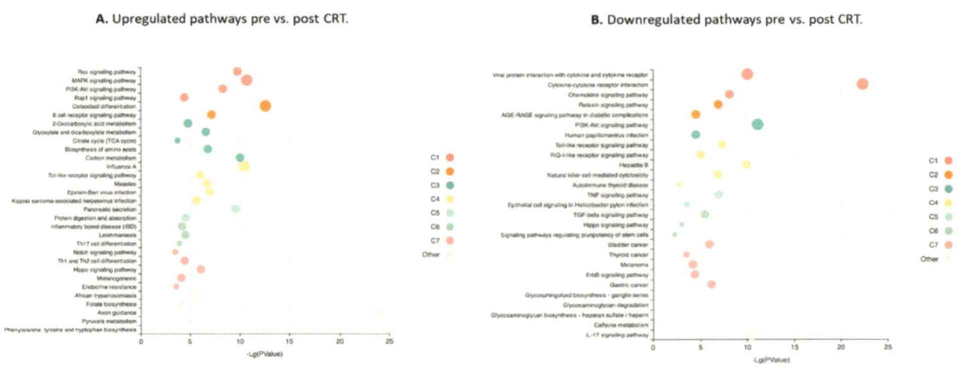

Figure 2.
KOBAS bubble plot of KEGG pathways enriched in the set of significantly differentially expressed proteins between pre-and post-treatment based on a paired t-test in GBM. (A). Upregulated genes. (B). Downregulated. The bubble size reflects the KOBAS hypergeometric test p-value broken into ranges. Colors reflect clusters of related pathways [18].

biopsy. Co-expression modules in WGCNA have been employed to link expression profile data to survival. Zhou et al. used TCGA expression profile data and clinical information to screen out genes related to the prognosis of GBM, dividing patients into high- and low-risk groups [15]. The biological processes identified using GO analysis were cell cycle but less intuitively progesterone-mediated oocyte maturation and oocyte meiosis related with CDCA5 and CDCA8 identified as genes of interest with expression levels related to overall survival. GSEA (Gene Set Enrichment Analysis) [16] is a computational technique that is also often employed, producing sets of genes based on a differential expression that allows ranking and calculation of enrichment scores that can then be connected to biological processes. Hypoxia risk signatures have been obtained using TCGA and CGGA for low-grade glioma (LGG) and GBM using GSEA [17].

There is currently no single database or bioinformatics analysis that is considered the gold standard, and thus, most studies employ several approaches in part to validate that the signals map to similar networks or pathways when using a dataset. Most studies employ proteogenomic data from TCGA and Clinical Proteomic Tumor Analysis Consortium (CPTAC) or examine original data in conjunction with repository data from public databases (**Table 2**).

Several barriers emerge in attributing meaning to molecular interaction networks, however. It is worthwhile noting that most published studies that aim to link clinical and omic data do so by leveraging several databases to filter and assign meaning to the measured signal. There is also significant concern that incorrect meaning may be attributed to molecule modification in different scenarios based on the malignancy studied, the treatment, and the tissue wherein the signal was obtained (**Figure 1**).

Author	Title	Sample / Technique	Clinical factors	Survival analysis	Time points
Lam KHB, et al. Nat Commun. 2022 Jan 10;13 [1]:116 [19].	Topographic mapping of the glioblastoma proteome reveals a triple-axis model of intra-tumoral heterogeneity.	20 patients Tumor tissue/Mass spectrometry	Age, sex, resection	No	One (tissue)
Duhamel M, et al. Nat Commun. 2022 Nov 4;13 [1]:6665 [20].	Spatial analysis of the glioblastoma proteome reveals specific molecular signatures and markers of survival.	96 patients 46 tumors analyzed mass spectrometry-based spatially-resolved proteomics guided by mass spectrometry imaging Integration of protein expression and clinical information, a 5-protein signature is associated with survival. The expression of these 5 proteins was validated by immunofluorescence on an additional cohort of 50 patients.	Age, sex, KPS, resection, tumor location, molecular features	Yes	One (tissue)

Author	Title	Sample / Technique	Clinical factors	Survival analysis	Time points
Rose M, et al. Front Immunol. 2021 Sep 27;12:746168 [21]	Surfaceome Proteomic of Glioblastoma Revealed Potential Targets for Immunotherapy.	Cell lines Proteins verified in patient GBM using spatial proteomic guided by MALDI-mass spectrometry	none	No	One (cell lines, tissue)
Syafruddin SE, et al. BMC Cancer. 2021 Jul 23;21 [1]:850 [22]	Integration of RNA-Seq and proteomics data identifies glioblastoma multiforme surfaceome signature.	RNA-Seq data from TCGA GBM (n = 166) and GTEx normal brain cortex (n = 408)	Age, sex, treatment	No	One (tissue)
Yanovich-Arad G, et al. Cell Rep. 2021 Mar 2;34 [10]:108787 [23].	Proteogenomics of glioblastoma associates molecular patterns with survival.	87 GBM patients high-resolution mass spectrometry proteomics and RNA sequencing (RNA-seq). Integrative analysis of protein expression, RNA expression, and patient clinical information	Age, sex, KPS, resection, tumor location, IDH status, treatment	Yes	One (tissue)
Wang LB et al. Cancer Cell. 2021 Apr 12;39 [4]: 509-528.e20 [24].	Clinical Proteomic Tumor Analysis Consortium. Proteogenomic and metabolomic characterization of human glioblastoma.	Integrated analysis of genomic, proteomic, post-translational modification, and metabolomic data on 99 treatment-naive GBMs	Age, sex, BMI, race, ethnicity, smoking history, tumor location	Yes	One (tissue)
Krauze AV et al. Frontiers in Oncology. Pending print [18]	Glioblastoma survival is associated with distinct proteomic alteration signatures post chemoirradiation in a large-scale proteomic panel.	Proteogenomic analysis pre vs. post chemoirradiation in 83 GBM patients	Age, sex, KPS. RPA, tumor location, resection, MGMT status, management, radiation volumes	Yes	Two Serum proteome pre and post-treatment

Table 2.
Major publications linking the GBM proteome to clinical factors.

Measurements augment this concern in specific settings with only one time point. The signals arrived at using the abovementioned studies are all largely distinct, given different data acquisition means, various data linkages, and analysis timing as databases evolve. This causes difficulty in biological understanding since few signals are common between studies, and novel markers are often not validated in independent cohorts and might not present an opportunity for validation due to difficulty in the sample acquisition (e.g., tumor tissue), cost, or limited sample available for multiple analyses. Lack of validation poses significant challenges. Thus results need to be interpreted cautiously since several alternative versions of the same linkage are conceivable (**Figure 1**), given additional published data. It is anticipated that as connections grow, the annotation will improve. However, the annotation will continue to be subject to bias as new clinical data and unidentified or unpublished markers will not link potentially missing meaningful biological connections that may not be reflected or surfaced in interaction databases and bioinformatics applications. This is augmented by the ambiguity of captured biological signals and attribution of differentially expressed signals to upregulated and downregulated signaling pathways (**Figure 2**), making interpretation difficult. The attribution of meaning to omic data will be discussed in the next section.

3. Attribution of meaning to omic data using proteogenomic analysis

The meaning assigned to novel signals along molecular networks can align with specific cells cell types, specific pathways, clinical aspects of the disease, or specific outcomes (**Table 2**). Increasingly studies link tissue culture, animal, and human data with outcomes data along molecular interaction networks. The attribution of meaning to omic data can be enhanced by connecting it to mechanistic roles via pathways (**Figure 2**), to other omic data (**Figure 3**), and to clinical features to elicit linkage to patient outcomes. Existing and established connections may be the result of data linked to a specific disease process or intervention or a novel scenario, such as the study of a novel intervention or agent. Additional connections can be based

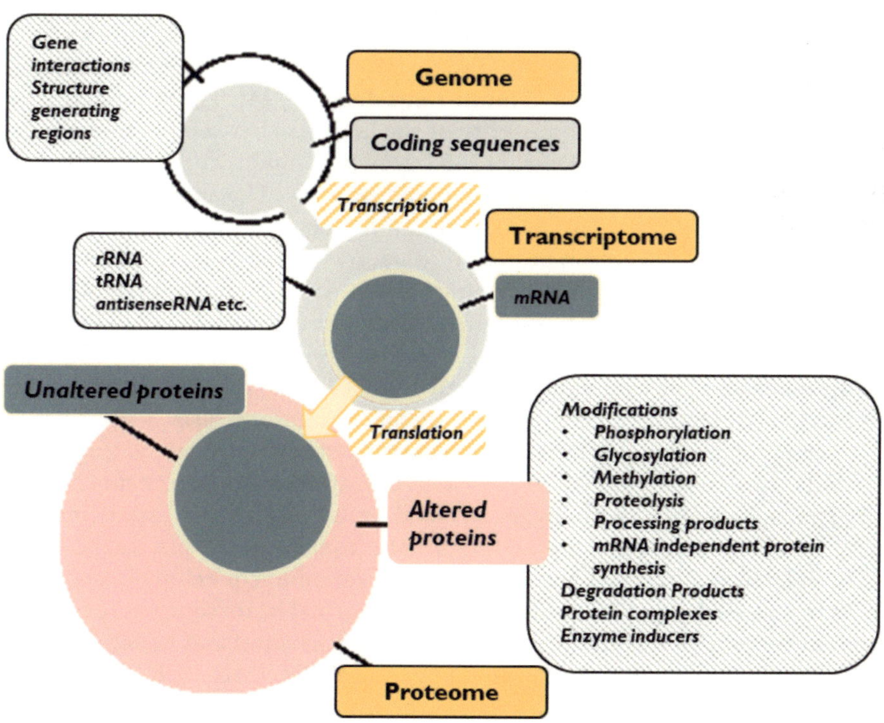

Figure 3.
The proteome results from gene expression and subsequent modification of resulting proteins. Filtration of the signal along the path from genome to transcriptome to proteome with transcription and then translation of information as mechanistic steps challenging linkages along molecular interaction networks [25].

on data sources such as imaging and pathology slides that involve data analysis based on structural or textural features. The previous section discussed tool sets linking largely undefined signals to molecular interaction pathways. The results of these analyses have added insight to our understanding of glioma heterogeneity. The work of Lam et al., using a liquid chromatography-tandem mass spectrometry (LC-MS/MS)-based proteomic analysis on tumor tissue to generate an atlas that connects the levels of 4794 proteins to hallmark histomorphologic niches to define intra-tumoral molecular patterns [19]. The proteomic patterns identified were based on anatomical niches aligning less strongly with the Verhaak signature [26] and were not included due to low concordance between protein and RNA. This study ultimately resulted in three groups defined by KRAS_targets, MYC_targets, and Hypoxia to define heterogeneity in GBM [19]. When comparing the groups to drug response employing 543 drugs in the CTRPv2 dataset to GBM cells grown in culture, heterogeneity was again observed but also diminished response based on hypoxia signatures with some differential response in MYC-enriched vs. KRAS-enriched acknowledging limitations of the study. Without the histological annotation, but rather using spectrometry-based spatially-resolved proteomics guided by mass spectrometry imaging, Duhamel et al. examined GBM heterogeneity in 46 tumors in relation to survival, resulting from arriving at three molecular groups associated with immune, neurogenesis, and tumorigenesis signatures [20]. The groups identified were, by contrast, not associated with unique histological areas. Group A (cluster 2) was associated with neuro-developmental genes, linked to neurogenesis and axon guidance; group B (cluster 1) with microglial activation, including iron transporters and proteins involved in coagulation, and group C (cluster 3) was associated with tumor growth. The authors concluded that heterogeneity is microenvironment-specific and presented a 21 gene signature and 5 proteins associated with survival. Two notable proteogenomic approaches have recently connected multi-omic data [23, 24]. These comprehensive data linkage studies reveal the complexity of the interplay between proteomic, transcriptomic, and genomic data. A recent MS-based proteomics and RNA-seq analysis identified molecular differences associated with survival. The analysis showcases the complexity of data linkage and difficulty in sample acquisition, which utilized 84 samples, 54 with high-resolution proteomic data, 65 with high-quality RNA-seq data, and 32 with both [23]. Given the importance of this data and the burden of disease in glioma, such a sample size illustrates the difficulties faced by the field in integrating omic analysis to arrive at meaningful and actionable conclusions. The identified proteomic modules were associated with survival, whereas the RNA modules did not, unless the IDH mutated samples were included in the analysis. A good correlation between proteomics and transcriptomics was noted in sex -correlating modules [23]. This data also linked increased fatty acid oxidation with shorter survival and oxidative phosphorylation with longer survival time. A subsequent study involving integrated proteogenomic and metabolomic data from 10 platforms, including RNA sequencing, DNA methylation arrays with whole genome sequencing investigating 99 GBMs from CPTAC and 10 unmatched GTEx normal brain samples revealed four immune subtypes with histone acetylation associations, lipid and metabolome profiles. The key signaling pathways that emerged were RTK/RAS, PI3K/AKT, and p53/cell cycle [24]. Dysregulation in signaling involving RTK, PI3K, WNT, and NOTCH pathways was present in all tumors with distinct drug connectivity analysis along EGFR and NF1 altered signatures. Another promising facet of analysis, given the relevance to druggable targets, is the surfaceome. Data from GBM cell lines examining the surfaceome with spatial proteomic-guided MALDI-mass spectrometry identified

87 overexpressed proteins, with 7 already in clinical trials and 3 of unknown interaction [21]. An integrated analysis of RNA-Seq data from TCGA and GTEx normal brain cortex databases was carried out to examine the surfaceome in GBM and identified 2381 dysregulated genes, of which 395 were surfaceome related, and a 6 gene signature was arrived at, including HLA-DRA, CD44, and SLC1A5, EGFR, ITGB2, PTPRJ with several clinically approved drugs potentially effective [22]. These studies take the large proteogenomic signals and arrive at pathways of significance that allow the classification of glioma. However, the connection to prognosis is inconsistent, and although there are mechanistic commonalities among studies, specific protein signals vary, with very few in common among studies. Existing or evolving pathways that may not yet map in molecular interaction pathways will require a referencing process to evolving data. This is embedded in several of the approaches in **Table 2**, using manual curation and proprietary linkages. In glioma, the most common linkages are made to hypoxia, angiogenesis, epithelial-mesenchymal transition, glioma stem cells, and the interplay of metabolism and immune response with these hallmarks of cancer. Because certain molecules are more widely studied and important data is present to draw from, such as p53 and EGFR, irrespective of the data input, p53 or EGFR will emerge as linkage centric. Sex differences have increasingly been studied in glioma, but specific classification via molecular interactions is evolving. Equally, there is no linkage along the lines of tumor burden with no omic signature of tumor burden currently defined. Some clinical characteristics of glioma are linked to glioma type and prognosis and thus present important avenues for classification, such as age at diagnosis, which correlates with the type of glioma and prognosis [27]. Novel proteins in any one malignancy will, however, map to networks wherein the protein has been described in another malignancy, limiting the ability to investigate its meaning in specific scenarios.

4. Emerging pathway and omic signatures in glioma

Pathways that have emerged in previous studies have been described in other studies and merit more in-depth analysis. Several, including Notch, NF-κB signaling, Ferroptosis, lipidome, fatty acid metabolism, stem cell propagation, evolution, and sustainment, appear more prominently and will be highlighted here. Notch has emerged in several recent proteogenomic analyses [18, 23, 24] as a potential mediator of glioma proliferation, invasion, stemness, and resistance to treatment [28, 29]. It has been connected to sex differences and response to treatment [30] and is a promising immunotherapy target [31]. Notch, possibly regulated through posttranslational modification, has been implicated in other cancers and linked to regulating multiple genes, including EGFR and NF-κB [32]. NF-κB has relationships to subunits linked to poorer outcomes at the RNA level and longer survival at the protein level, while Notch signaling was tumor-promoting overall [18, 23] with evolving directionality with respect to the protein level. Ferroptosis, a novel mechanism of cell death, has been increasingly described in glioma with connections to the lipidome and known mediators, including p53 and MAPK, and iron metabolism [33, 34]. It is increasingly associated with adaptive resistance mechanisms and may be employed in future therapeutic avenues [35]. Given the connection to iron metabolism, ferroptosis-based interactions in proteogenomic analysis via heme signaling and peroxisome classifications [18, 36, 37]. Several agents, including temozolomide, target ferroptosis [38]. Its links to the lipidome will likely benefit from increasing analysis as connections between the metabolome and the lipidome and tumor resistance are growing in glioma. Fatty acid metabolism is of increasing interest for multiple reasons. Gliomas have an increased level of lipid content as compared to normal tissues, and the brain has a higher lipid content than other tissues, making the lipidome an exciting avenue of research since it can allow for the classification of omic signal [39]. The lipidome is liked to radiation resistance [40] and metabolism, including relationships to IDH mutation, EGFR, PTEN, and MGMT promoter mutation via association with alterations in lipid metabolism [41]. Stem cells as mediators of treatment resistance have been an essential facet of glioma research and have now been connected to virtually every signaling pathway. In their histomorphologic niche analysis, Lam et al. found that the infiltrating tumor region was associated with both neuronal systems and stem cell-related pathways [19], while another proteogenomic study identified a cluster related to the regulation of stem cell maintenance [23]. Lower survival in glioma has been linked to stem cell burden [18, 23]. Still, there is currently no robust stem cell signature in part because the formation and sustainment of stem cells are deeply linked to the microenvironment, metabolism, and adaptive resistance, fostering heterogeneity and is also a dynamic process that is only partially captured in single time point, single tissue sample analyses [42].

5. Tumor biology and treatment strategies in glioma

Despite the data proliferation in the glioma, including its analysis along genomic, transcriptomic, and proteomic data sets now extending over 10 years [43], management has remained the same. Typical management is still comprised of maximal safe resection followed by concurrent chemoirradiation and adjuvant temozolomide. Tumor failure ensues almost universally, and upon recurrence, rarely management, including chemotherapy and re-irradiation, results in relatively limited benefit. The use of additional agents to the standard of care has yet to significantly improve outcomes and is implemented on trial with no standard of care agent yet to be implemented. Meanwhile, only 10% of patients benefit from genomic analysis.

Molecular subtypes based on RNA sequencing have not been connected to prognosis and have become challenging to connect to other omic data based on clinical samples [26, 44]. Biomarkers for response and resistance are lacking, and prognostic markers have struggled to reach predictive roles [45]. Criteria such as REMARK (Reporting Recommendations for Tumor Marker Prognostic Studies) have needed to be more consistently implemented, and a plethora of emerging markers are difficult to conceptualize for inclusion in clinical trials [46]. As a result, emerging novel agents had theoretical backing for biological mechanisms of action that should have translated into clinical benefit, but limited benefit emerged for multiple reasons.

Several targets and approaches predominate. EGFR has been extensively studied since it is the receptor tyrosine kinase most amplified in glioma. However, its mechanistic implications remain unclear, and despite several attempts at targeting EGFR in clinical trials, no significant outcome benefits have been obtained. This is likely multifactorial, including tumor heterogeneity and a variety of mechanisms for EGFR activation, which is complex with both overexpression of the receptor and ligand production [47]. Therapeutic attempts have included tyrosine kinase inhibitors (Erlotinib, Gefitinib, Lapatinib, Osimertinib), monoclonal antibodies (Cetuximab), immunotherapy (CAR-T cells targeting EGFRvIII) and others. There are several possible reasons for the lack of benefit noted, including tumor heterogeneity and the wide-ranging signaling that occurs downstream of genetic EGFR alterations that can lead to resistance and phenotypic diversity. There is also no specific biomarker that defines possible responses to EGFR-mediated interventions. IDH1 and 2 mutations have also been widely studied and are an integral component of glioma classification, given the association with prognosis [48]. The 2021 classification of glioma includes IDH alteration to separate low-grade and high-grade gliomas that are IDH mutated from GBM, which is IDH-wildtype [49]. It should be noted that existing data does not yet reflect this classification, and IDH status in most glioma cohorts does not yet include IDH status, although this is likely to change as more data emerges [50]. The mechanism by which IDH mutation, which is common in lower-grade gliomas and uncommon in GBM, results in superior outcomes is unclear. IDH mutation impacts tumor growth by inhibiting glutaminase and altering metabolism [51]; however, IDH mutation also fosters the hypermethylation phenotype with potentially conflicting results for clinical therapeutic interventions [52]. Targeting the IDH mutation is evolving with recent data in this space [53]. In a double-blind phase 3 trial, Vorasidenib, an inhibitor of mutant IDH1 and IDH2 enzymes, improved progression-free survival and delayed the time to intervention in patients with grade II IDH mutated glioma. There are currently 475 interventional recruiting trials in glioma. Thus, it is anticipated that this data growth, matched by biospecimen acquisition and accompanied by biomarkers, will increasingly define the mechanisms of resistance and response in glioma to link biology and treatment strategies. Potentially actionable biomarkers, however, are evaluated based on clinically associated prognosis, which can be based on outdated endpoints. Progression is based on Response Assessment in Neuro-Oncology (RANO) criteria that include no omic signatures or relationships [54]. Imaging features that have evolved to integrate computational analysis are equally not currently included [55–58]. The rapid evolution of computational approaches and their application should be vetted for interpretability through a clinical lens. Intersectional clinical and computational expertise is needed to link omics, molecular interactions, and clinical data to address the missing link between tumor biology and treatment strategies. Expertise that functions at the intersection of computational approaches and medicine is on the rise and should be included when new trials are designed and implemented to harness maximal data output for future analyses.

6. Conclusions

Molecular interaction databases and bioinformatics applications have been growing in number and usage to identify novel signals in glioma and annotate emerging data. However, challenges remain, including basing conclusions on any type of biospecimen, time point, or intervention and lack of transparency as to how linkages in bioinformatics platforms were generated. Emerging signals are primarily distinct from one another given different data acquisition means, various data linkages, and analysis timing as databases evolve. This causes difficulty in biological understanding since few signals are shared between studies and novel markers are often not validated in independent cohorts. Results are growing and perpetuate inclusion into databases but can generate circular connections, which need to be interpreted cautiously since several alternative versions of the same linkage are conceivable given additional published data and validation. As associations grow, the annotation will improve but can be subject to bias as new clinical data and unidentified or unpublished markers will remain unlinked. Biologic signal ambiguity in the attribution of differentially expressed signals to upregulated and downregulated signaling pathways is the subject of ongoing studies, and thus directionality of signal change is evolving. Endpoints employed to study large-scale omic data need to be updated to reflect potentially actionable biomarkers, and intersectional expertise needs to be implemented in clinical trials to allow for future data integration and analysis.

Conflict of interest

The authors declare no conflict of interest.

Abbreviations

CGGA	Chinese Glioma Genome Atlas
COG	Clusters of Orthologous Genes
CPTAC	Clinical Proteomic Tumor Analysis Consortium
GBM	Glioblastoma
GEO	Gene Expression Omnibus
GO	Gene Ontology
IPA	Ingenuity Pathway Analysis
KEGG	Kyoto Encyclopedia of Genes and Genomes
KOBAS	KEGG Orthology-Based Annotation System
LGG	Low-Grade Glioma
MGMT	O6-Methylguanine-DNA Methyltransferase
MSigDB	The Molecular Signatures Database
RANO	Response Assessment in Neuro-Oncology
REMARK	Reporting Recommendations for Tumor Marker Prognostic Studies
ssGSEA	Single-sample Gene Set Enrichment Analysis
STRING	Search Tool for the Retrieval of Interacting Genes/Proteins
TCGA	The Cancer Genome Atlas
WGCNA	Weighted Gene Co-expression Network Analysis

Author details

Andra V. Krauze
National Cancer Institute, NIH, Bethesda, MD, USA

*Address all correspondence to: andra.krauze@nih.gov

References

[1] Krämer A, Green J, Pollard J Jr, Tugendreich S. Causal analysis approaches in ingenuity pathway analysis. Bioinformatics. 2014;**30**(4):523-530

[2] von Mering C, Huynen M, Jaeggi D, Schmidt S, Bork P, Snel B. String: A database of predicted functional associations between proteins. Nucleic Acids Research. 2003;**31**(1):258-261

[3] Kanehisa M, Sato Y, Kawashima M. KEGG mapping tools for uncovering hidden features in biological data. Protein Science. 2022;**31**(1):47-53

[4] AV. K. Web of Science Search: Web of Science. 2023. Available from: https://www.webofscience.com/.

[5] Slidesgo. Healthcare Infographics Slidesgo 2022 [Human Icon and Test Tube Icon]. Available from: https://slidesgo.com/theme/healthcare-infographics#search-healthcare&position-1&results-35

[6] Szklarczyk D, Gable AL, Nastou KC, Lyon D, Kirsch R, Pyysalo S, et al. The STRING database in 2021: Customizable protein–protein networks and functional characterization of user-uploaded gene/measurement sets. Nucleic Acids Research. 2020;**49**:D605-DD12

[7] Li Y, Deng G, Qi Y, Zhang H, Gao L, Jiang H, et al. Bioinformatic profiling of prognosis-related genes in malignant glioma microenvironment. Medical Science Monitor. 2020;**26**:e924054

[8] Mischkulnig M, Kiesel B, Rötzer-Pejrimovsky T, Borkovec M, Lang A, Millesi M, et al. The impact of heme biosynthesis regulation on glioma aggressiveness: Correlations with diagnostic molecular markers. Frontiers in Molecular Neuroscience. 2022;**15**:928355

[9] Güven E, Afzal M, Kazmi I. Screening the significant hub genes by comparing tumor cells, normoxic and hypoxic glioblastoma stem-like cell lines using Co-expression analysis in glioblastoma. Genes (Basel). 15 Mar 2022;**13**(3):518

[10] Li J, Zhang Z, Guo K, Wu S, Guo C, Zhang X, et al. Identification of a key glioblastoma candidate gene, FUBP3, based on weighted gene co-expression network analysis. BMC Neurology. 2022;**22**(1):139

[11] Ghosh S, Dutta S, Thorne G, Boston A, Barfield A, Banerjee N, et al. Core canonical pathways involved in developing human glioblastoma multiforme (GBM). International Journal of Scientific Research in Science, Engineering and Technology. 2017;**3**(1):458-465

[12] Tasci E, Jagasia S, Zhuge Y, Sproull M, Cooley-Zgela T, Mackey M, et al. RadWise: A rank-based hybrid feature weighting and selection method for proteomic categorization of Chemoirradiation in patients with glioblastoma. Cancers. 2023;**15**:2672

[13] Langfelder P, Horvath S. WGCNA: An R package for weighted correlation network analysis. BMC Bioinformatics. 2008;**9**(1):559

[14] Yang Q, Wang R, Wei B, Peng C, Wang L, Hu G, et al. Candidate biomarkers and molecular mechanism investigation for glioblastoma multiforme utilizing WGCNA. BioMed Research International. 2018;**2018**:4246703

[15] Zhou J, Guo H, Liu L, Hao S, Guo Z, Zhang F, et al. Construction of co-expression modules related to survival by WGCNA and identification of potential prognostic biomarkers in glioblastoma. Journal of Cellular and Molecular Medicine. 2021;**25**(3):1633-1644

[16] Subramanian A, Tamayo P, Mootha VK, Mukherjee S, Ebert BL, Gillette MA, et al. Gene set enrichment analysis: A knowledge-based approach for interpreting genome-wide expression profiles. Proceedings of the National Academy of Sciences of the United States of America. 2005;**102**(43):15545-15550

[17] Lin W, Wu S, Chen X, Ye Y, Weng Y, Pan Y, et al. Characterization of hypoxia signature to evaluate the tumor immune microenvironment and predict prognosis in glioma groups. Frontiers in Oncology. 2020;**10**:796

[18] Krauze AV, Sierk M, Nguyen T, Chen Q, Yan C, Hu Y, et al. Glioblastoma survival is associated with distinct proteomic alteration signatures post chemoirradiation in a large-scale proteomic panel. Frontiers in Oncology. 10 Aug 2023;**13**:1127645

[19] Lam KHB, Leon AJ, Hui W, Lee SC-E, Batruch I, Faust K, et al. Topographic mapping of the glioblastoma proteome reveals a triple-axis model of intra-tumoral heterogeneity. Nature Communications. 2022;**13**(1):116

[20] Duhamel M, Drelich L, Wisztorski M, Aboulouard S, Gimeno JP, Ogrinc N, et al. Spatial analysis of the glioblastoma proteome reveals specific molecular signatures and markers of survival. Nature Communications. 2022;**13**(1):6665

[21] Rose M, Cardon T, Aboulouard S, Hajjaji N, Kobeissy F, Duhamel M, et al. Surfaceome proteomic of glioblastoma revealed potential targets for immunotherapy. Frontiers in Immunology. 2021;**12**:746168

[22] Syafruddin SE, Nazarie W, Moidu NA, Soon BH, Mohtar MA. Integration of RNA-Seq and proteomics data identifies glioblastoma multiforme surfaceome signature. BMC Cancer. 2021;**21**(1):850

[23] Yanovich-Arad G, Ofek P, Yeni E, Mardamshina M, Danilevsky A, Shomron N, et al. Proteogenomics of glioblastoma associates molecular patterns with survival. Cell Reports. 2021;**34**(9):108787

[24] Wang LB, Karpova A, Gritsenko MA, Kyle JE, Cao S, Li Y, et al. Proteogenomic and metabolomic characterization of human glioblastoma. Cancer Cell. 2021;**39**(4):509-28.e20

[25] Caspardavid. Das Proteom als Resultat der Genexpression und nachfolgenden Modifikation der entstandenen Proteinmoleküle. Wikimedia Commons: Wikimedia Commons; 2005. Available from: https://commons.wikimedia.org/wiki/File:Proteom.png [Accessed: January 9, 2005]

[26] Verhaak RGW, Hoadley KA, Purdom E, Wang V, Qi Y, Wilkerson MD, et al. Integrated genomic analysis identifies clinically relevant subtypes of glioblastoma characterized by abnormalities in PDGFRA, IDH1, EGFR, and NF1. Cancer Cell. 2010;**17**(1):98-110

[27] Kaubryte J, Lai AG. Pan-cancer prognostic genetic mutations and clinicopathological factors associated with survival outcomes: A systematic review. NPJ Precision Oncology. 2022;**6**(1):27

[28] Parmigiani E, Taylor V, Giachino C. Oncogenic and tumor-suppressive

functions of NOTCH Signaling in glioma. Cell. 15 Oct 2020;**9**(10):2304

[29] Yahyanejad S, Theys J, Vooijs M. Targeting Notch to overcome radiation resistance. Oncotarget. 2016;**7**(7):7610-7628

[30] Giuli MV, Mancusi A, Giuliani E, Screpanti I, Checquolo S. Notch signaling in female cancers: A multifaceted node to overcome drug resistance. Cancer Drug Resistance. 2021;**4**(4):805-836

[31] Li X, Yan X, Wang Y, Kaur B, Han H, Yu J. The Notch signaling pathway: A potential target for cancer immunotherapy. Journal of Hematology & Oncology. 2023;**16**(1):45

[32] D'Amico M, De Amicis F. Aberrant Notch signaling in gliomas: A potential landscape of actionable converging targets for combination approach in therapies resistance. Cancer Drug Resistance. 2022;**5**(4):939-953

[33] Wan S, Zhang G, Liu R, Abbas MN, Cui H. Pyroptosis, ferroptosis, and autophagy cross-talk in glioblastoma opens up new avenues for glioblastoma treatment. Cell Communication and Signaling. 2023;**21**(1):115

[34] Shi J, Yang N, Han M, Qiu C. Emerging roles of ferroptosis in glioma. Frontiers in Oncology. 2022;**12**:993316

[35] de Souza I, Ramalho MCC, Guedes CB, Osawa IYA, Monteiro LKS, Gomes LR, et al. Ferroptosis modulation: Potential therapeutic target for glioblastoma treatment. International Journal of Molecular Sciences. 21 Jun 2022;**23**(13):6879

[36] Kim JA. Peroxisome Metabolism in Cancer. Cells. 2020;**9**:7

[37] Tang D, Kroemer G. Peroxisome: The new player in ferroptosis. Signal Transduction and Targeted Therapy. 2020;**5**(1):273

[38] Zhou Y, Fang C, Xu H, Yuan L, Liu Y, Wang X, et al. Ferroptosis in glioma treatment: Current situation, prospects, and drug applications. Frontiers in Oncology. 2022;**12**:989896

[39] Guo D, Bell EH, Chakravarti A. Lipid metabolism emerges as a promising target for malignant glioma therapy. CNS Oncology. 2013;**2**(3):289-299

[40] Jiang N, Xie B, Xiao W, Fan M, Xu S, Duan Y, et al. Fatty acid oxidation fuels glioblastoma radioresistance with CD47-mediated immune evasion. Nature Communications. 2022;**13**(1):1511

[41] El Khayari A, Bouchmaa N, Taib B, Wei Z, Zeng A, El Fatima R. Metabolic rewiring in glioblastoma cancer: EGFR, IDH, and beyond. Frontiers in Oncology. 2022;**12**:901951

[42] Dirkse A, Golebiewska A, Buder T, Nazarov PV, Muller A, Poovathingal S, et al. Stem cell-associated heterogeneity in glioblastoma results from intrinsic tumor plasticity shaped by the microenvironment. Nature Communications. 2019;**10**(1):1787

[43] Brennan CW, Verhaak RG, McKenna A, Campos B, Noushmehr H, Salama SR, et al. The somatic genomic landscape of glioblastoma. Cell. 2013;**155**(2):462-477

[44] Vaubel RA, Tian S, Remonde D, Schroeder MA, Mladek AC, Kitange GJ, et al. Genomic and phenotypic characterization of a broad panel of patient-derived xenografts reflects the diversity of glioblastoma. Clinical Cancer Research. 2020;**26**(5):1094-1104

[45] Mansouri A, Hachem LD, Mansouri S, Nassiri F, Laperriere NJ,

Xia D, et al. MGMT promoter methylation status testing to guide therapy for glioblastoma: Refining the approach based on emerging evidence and current challenges. Neuro-Oncology. 2019;**21**(2):167-178

[46] Altman DG, McShane LM, Sauerbrei W, Taube SE. Reporting recommendations for tumor marker prognostic studies (REMARK): Explanation and elaboration. BMC Medicine. 2012;**10**(1):51

[47] Oprita A, Baloi SC, Staicu GA, Alexandru O, Tache DE, Danoiu S, et al. Updated insights on EGFR signaling pathways in glioma. International Journal of Molecular Sciences. 8 Jan 2021;**22**(2):587

[48] Han S, Liu Y, Cai SJ, Qian M, Ding J, Larion M, et al. IDH mutation in glioma: Molecular mechanisms and potential therapeutic targets. British Journal of Cancer. 2020;**122**(11):1580-1589

[49] Louis DN, Perry A, Wesseling P, Brat DJ, Cree IA, Figarella-Branger D, et al. The 2021 WHO classification of tumors of the central nervous system: A summary. Neuro-Oncology. 2021;**23**(8):1231-1251

[50] Zakharova G, Efimov V, Raevskiy M, Rumiantsev P, Gudkov A, Belogurova-Ovchinnikova O, et al. Reclassification of TCGA diffuse glioma profiles linked to transcriptomic, epigenetic, genomic and clinical data, according to the 2021 WHO CNS tumor classification. International Journal of Molecular Sciences. 21 Dec 2022;**24**(1):157

[51] Seltzer MJ, Bennett BD, Joshi AD, Gao P, Thomas AG, Ferraris DV, et al. Inhibition of glutaminase preferentially slows the growth of glioma cells with mutant IDH1. Cancer Research. 2010;**70**(22):8981-8987

[52] Kayabolen A, Yilmaz E, Bagci-Onder T. IDH mutations in glioma: Double-edged sword in clinical applications? Biomedicines. 10 Jul 2021;**9**(7):799

[53] Mellinghoff IK, van den Bent MJ, Blumenthal DT, Touat M, Peters KB, Clarke J, et al. Vorasidenib in IDH1- or IDH2-mutant low-grade glioma. The New England Journal of Medicine. 17 Aug 2023;**389**(7):589-601

[54] Soffietti R, Bettegowda C, Mellinghoff IK, Warren KE, Ahluwalia MS, De Groot JF, et al. Liquid biopsy in gliomas: A RANO review and proposals for clinical applications. Neuro-Oncology. 2022;**24**(6):855-871

[55] Bakas S, Sako C, Akbari H, Bilello M, Sotiras A, Shukla G, et al. The University of Pennsylvania glioblastoma (UPenn-GBM) cohort: Advanced MRI, clinical, genomics, & radiomics. Scientific Data. 2022;**9**(1):453

[56] Jia X, Zhai Y, Song D, Wang Y, Wei S, Yang F, et al. A multiparametric MRI-based radiomics nomogram for preoperative prediction of survival stratification in glioblastoma patients with standard treatment. Frontiers in Oncology. 2022;**12**:758622

[57] Habib A, Jovanovich N, Hoppe M, Ak M, Mamindla P, R Colen R, et al. MRI-based radiomics and radiogenomics in the management of low-grade Gliomas: Evaluating the evidence for a paradigm shift. Journal of Clinical Medicine. 1 Apr 2021;**10**(7):1411

[58] Lohmann P, Galldiks N, Kocher M, Heinzel A, Filss CP, Stegmayr C, et al. Radiomics in neuro-oncology: Basics, workflow, and applications. Methods. 2021;**188**:112-121

Chapter 3

Role of miRNA in Glioma Pathogenesis, Diagnosis, and Therapeutic Outcomes

Manendra Singh Tomar and Ashutosh Shrivastava

Abstract

Glioma is the most aggressive tumor of glial cells in the brain and spinal cord. It comprises 30% of all brain tumors. Even in the presence of current multimodal therapeutic regimens, the life expectancy of more than 2 years is very rare. MicroRNAs (miRNAs) are short, non-coding RNAs produced naturally in the body and control gene expression. Many evidence-based hypotheses show that miRNA expression is aberrantly influenced in glioma due to amplification or deletion of miRNA genes, inappropriate transcriptional regulation of miRNAs, dysregulated epigenetic alterations, or faults in the miRNA biogenesis machinery. In some circumstances, miRNAs promote tumorigenesis, whereas under other circumstances, they can act as tumor suppressors in glioma. In gliomas, miRNA is involved in cell proliferation signaling, evasion of growth suppressors, resistance to cell death, tumor cell infiltration, metastasis, and angiogenesis. More and more research is pointing to miRNAs as prospective biomarkers for glioma diagnosis, prognosis, and treatment targets or tools; however, these claims have yet to be validated. Here, we discuss the role of microRNAs (miRNAs) as tumor suppressors and oncogenes in the growth of glioma.

Keywords: MiRNA, glioma, carcinogenesis, diagnostic biomarkers, therapeutics

1. Introduction

Gliomas are the primary brain neoplasm of the central nervous system (CNS) hypothesized to develop from neuroglial stem or progenitor cells. They have histologically been categorized as astrocytic, oligodendroglial, or ependymal tumors based on their histological appearance and accordingly given WHO categories I–IV, which indicate varying degrees of aggressiveness [1]. Due to the advent of new prognostic markers of glioma, WHO updated their classification based on new molecular markers in 2016 [2, 3]. Glioblastoma multiforme (GBM) has a high degree of lethality and low median survival of ~15 months after the initial diagnosis and the five-year survival is less than 10% [4]. The centerpiece of GBM treatment is surgery, followed by radiation and adjuvant chemotherapy. The blood-brain barrier (BBB) severely restricts therapeutic agent delivery to the CNS. Therefore, the accessibility of the drug to the tumor sites is the main obstacle for the development of new therapeutics for GBM [5]. Temozolomide (TMZ) is a first-choice alkylating agent inducted as a standard therapy for glioblastoma multiforme (GBM) and astrocytoma. TMZ has limited efficacy due to the development of intrinsic and extrinsic drug resistance in glioma [6].

Growing shreds of evidence suggest that microRNA (miRNA) has a role in the onset and progression of gliomas [7]. miRNAs were first identified in the nematode *Caenorhabditis elegans* but have now been detected in almost every eukaryotic organism. MicroRNA is postulated to influence around 30% of human genes that code for proteins and make up 1–5% of the human genome [8]. These are short, evolutionarily conserved, single-stranded, non-coding RNA molecules that bind the target mRNA and inhibit protein generation [8]. Thus, it is not surprising that numerous miRNAs with a function in controlling apoptosis have also been connected to the emergence and development of cancer and other neoplastic diseases. Half of all the miRNAs found in genomic regions are often altered or amplified in malignant tumors [9]. Moreover, miRNAs have been linked to many aspects of carcinogenesis, including their invasiveness, DNA repair, and acquired resistance. Due to their numerous functions, miRNAs could replace other classes of molecules as primary targets of therapy for glioma [10]. Different miRNAs have opposing roles as tumor suppressors and oncogenes. Moreover, signaling that promotes chemotherapy resistance and tumor promotion in glioma is also triggered by the alteration or overexpression of oncogenic miRNAs and the downregulation of tumor-suppressing miRNAs [11]. In addition to providing a bad prognosis for glioma, recent research found that cytosine methylation of mature miRNA decreases its tumor-suppressive ability [12].

Continued research on miRNA is critical to understand its functional role in early diagnosis and treatment of GBM. This book chapter provides an overview of the pivotal role of miRNAs in glioma development, with special emphasis on their function as a diagnostic biomarker and their therapeutic potential.

2. MicroRNA biogenesis

The biogenesis of miRNA is classified into canonical and non-canonical pathways [13]. Most of the miRNAs are processed using the well-established canonical biogenesis mechanism. The microprocessor complex, comprised of the RNA-binding protein DiGeorge Syndrome Critical Region 8 (DGCR8) and the ribonuclease III enzyme Drosha, converts pri-miRNAs generated from their genes into pre-miRNAs [14]. DGCR8 recognizes N [6] methyl adenosine mark, a type of post-transcriptional modification that promotes the initiation of miRNA biogenesis [15]. RNase III enzyme DROSHA recognizes and cleaves miRNA hairpins, resulting in the release of pre-miRNAs, *i.e.,* miRNAs with a length of 60–80 nucleotides [16]. The GTP-binding nuclear protein Ran (RanGTP)/exportin-5 (XPO5) complex transports pre-miRNAs from the nucleus to the cytoplasm, where Dicer processes them into mature miRNAs with functional and regulatory capabilities (**Figure 1**) [17]. Generally, mature miRNA has one guide strand and the other passenger strand. Next, an argonaute protein takes the miRNA duplex and forms a structure called the miRNA-Induced Silencing Complex (RISC) [18]. The RISC is a multiprotein complex that contains a single strand of miRNA. RISC acts as a template for the recognition of complementary mRNA based on the miRNA. Upon recognizing a matching strand, it triggers RNase and cleaves the RNA [19].

Non-canonical pathways begin with shRNA being cleaved by the microprocessor complex and then exported to the cytoplasm through the Exportin5/RanGTP complex.

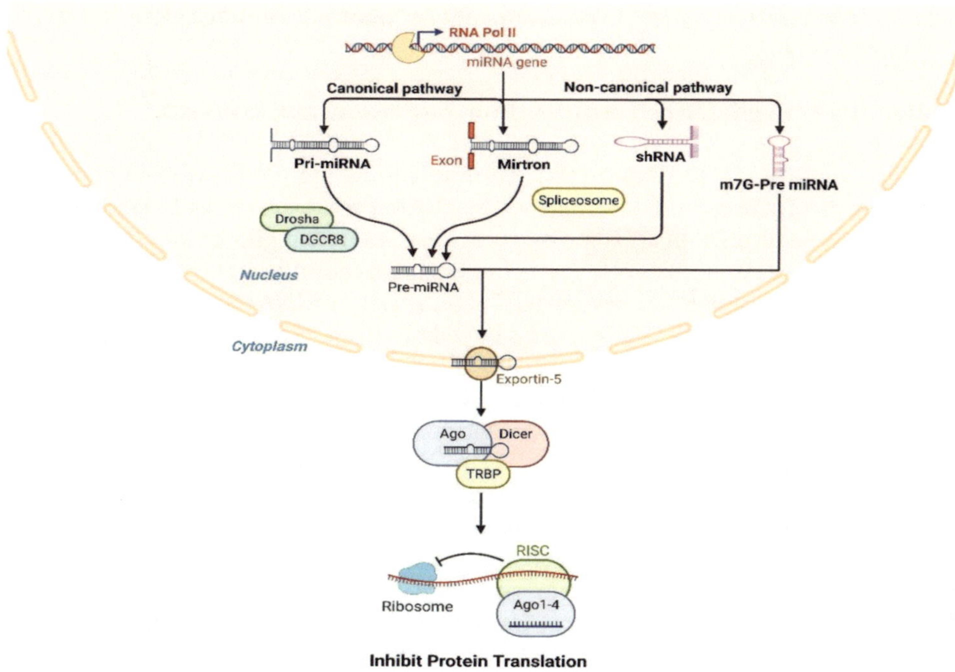

Figure 1.
Canonical and non-canonical pathway of miRNA biogenesis.

They undergo further processing that requires Argonaute 2 (AGO2) but does not need Dicer [20]. AGO2 is an RNA-binding protein that plays a crucial role in RNA-silencing processes. It regulates chromatin structure, transcriptional gene control, and RNA splicing, and plays a critical role in the development and function of microRNAs [21]. Two different types of miRNAs are processed through the non-canonical pathway. One of them, called mirtrons, is generated from an mRNA intron during the splicing process and the other is pre-miRNA that is capped with 7-methylguanosine (m7G) [20, 22]. A functioning miRISC complex is the endpoint of all possible routes that bind to mRNA and leads to translational inhibition (**Figure 1**) [23].

3. MicroRNA in the pathogenesis of glioma

Over the last several decades, researchers have worked hard to catalog miRNAs with aberrant expression patterns in glioma and choose the most promising ones for further evaluation as potential therapeutic targets. Multiple studies have shown a wide variety of miRNAs that play important roles in gliomas [24]. Ten signature miRNAs were described through TCGA analysis of mRNA expression data that may be crucial to distinguish between low- and high-risk GBM patients. Three of which were tumor-suppressing (miRNA-20a, miRNA-106a, and miRNA-17-5p), and seven of which were oncogenic (miRNA-31, miRNA-222, miRNA-148a, miRNA-221, miRNA-146b, miRNA-200b, and miRNA-193a) [25]. A significant proportion of miRNAs were observed to be overexpressed in glioma compared to normal brain tissue, 95 have relatively lower expression, and inconsistent findings were detected for 17 miRNAs [26].

3.1 MicroRNAs in glioma cell proliferation, migration, and invasion

Tumor-suppressing miRNAs are progressively linked to the advancement of anti-tumor treatment, *via* remodeling gene networks that are dysregulated in malignant tumors. The role of miRNA-21 is most extensively studied in glioma and is consistently upregulated. It inhibits cell death and boosts tumor invasion. It performs a role in chemo- and radiation resistance [27]. Similarly, miRNA-138 is one of the most significant miRNAs in GBM patients and correlates inversely with CD44 expression. Also, cell cycle arrest happens in GBM cells after overexpression or administration of miRNA-138, which negatively affects the expression of CD44 by directly binding to its 3′ UTR [28]. Highly expressed and exceptionally abundant miRNAs are found in glioma associated-human mesenchymal stem cells (GA-hMSCs)-derived exosomes, and one of them, miR-1587, has been shown to dramatically boost Glioma Stem Cell proliferation and clonogenicity. Exosomes generated from GA-hMSCs carry miR-1587 and cause the downregulation of tumor suppressor nuclear receptor corepressor NCOR1 resulting in the increased aggressiveness of GBM [29]. Additionally, miRNA-3620-5p enhances tumor cell proliferation and promotes stemness in glioma [30]. A Phosphatase and Tensin homolog (PTEN) regulating miRNA-26a is amplified in high-grade glioma and promotes tumor generation [31].

Other classes of miRNAs are also reported whose upregulation suppresses tumor cell proliferation such as miRNA-1825. This miRNA was found to be decreased in GBM patients, whereas its upregulation suppresses tumor progression by targeting CDK-14 through the Wnt/β-catenin signaling pathway [32]. According to another study, miRNA-10a regulates Wnt/β-catenin signaling and induces tumor generation via targeting myotubularin-related protein 3 [33]. In glioma tissues, decreased levels of miRNA-382-5p significantly increased the proliferation, invasion, and migration of tumor cells. Conversely, the transfer of mimics of miRNA-382-5p significantly decreases neoplasm formation as well as epithelial-to-mesenchymal transition (EMT) [34]. It has been established that the EMT plays a crucial role in the spread of tumors. The miRNA-16 suppresses EMT mainly through the downregulation of p-FAK and p-Akt expression and NF-kB and slug transcriptional activity [35].

During tumorigenesis, many proteolytic enzymes, including matrix metalloproteinases (MMPs), are overexpressed. Their job is to dissolve and degrade the matrix proteins of the surrounding normal brain tissue, which act as a barrier to migration and invasion of tumor cells [36]. Compared to healthy controls, glioma patients express more MMP-9. Further studies revealed that the expression status of MMP-9 and miRNA-34a was inversely correlated. Overexpression of miRNA-34a suppressed cell proliferation and migration in human glioma cells by MMP-9 [37]. Moreover, in GBM, miRNA-25 is elevated, and its expression levels correlate strongly with disease progression. miRNA-25 silencing significantly reduces tumor cell movement and invasiveness, by increasing the expression of cell adhesion molecule 2 (CADM2). This establishes CADM2 as a suitable target for miRNA-25 since CADM2 is dramatically downregulated in glioma [38]. On the other hand, miR-146b-5p, a tumor-suppressing miRNA, has been shown to have a negative correlation with its target gene MMP16. Glioma cells exhibit considerably lower amounts of miR-146b-5p, while simultaneously displaying higher levels of MMP16. The excessive production of miR-146b-5p also facilitates the disintegration of mRNA associated with MMP16 as well as restored miRNA action against glioma cell migration and invasion [39].

Cancer patients also have abnormal TGF-β signaling, and this abnormal signaling likely plays a role in the development and progression of several malignancies, including glioma [40]. A correlation study showed a positive relationship between TGF-β concentration and miRNA-132 mRNA levels. Additionally, it is reported that miRNA-132 specifically targets SMAD7 3'-UTR, resulting in downregulation of SMAD7 expression and modification of the TGF-β signaling pathway. Patients with glioma have an inverse relationship between miRNA-132 and SMAD7 [41]. Degradation or lower level of SMAD7 promotes autophagy-induced EMT and chemoresistance in glioma [42]. Evidence from these investigations shows that aberrant miRNA expression has a major role in tumor cell growth, migration, and invasion. All these findings strengthen the case for miRNAs as a potential therapeutic target in glioma.

3.2 MicroRNAs and angiogenesis network in glioma

The development of GBM is reliant on the establishment of new blood vessels since gliomas are highly vascularized tumors [43]. In response to various stimuli, vascular endothelial cells (ECs) proliferate, migrate, and differentiate to form new blood vessels, a process known as angiogenesis [44]. More intriguing is the discovery of miRNAs regulating angiogenesis *via* necessary biochemical pathways and its activation and/or inhibition. These miRNAs are known as "angiomiRs," and they play important functions in regulating the vascular network characteristics of gliomas [30].

Primary tumor endothelial cells of glioma have higher miR-296 levels than normal brain cells. Growth factor-induced miR-296 directly targets the hepatocyte growth factor-regulated tyrosine kinase substrate (HGS) mRNA, decreasing HGS levels and reducing HGS-mediated degradation of the growth factor receptors VEGFR2 and PDGFR-β. This activates angiogenesis in glioma cells [45]. Also, dysregulation of miRNA-24 in glioma cells promotes microvascular proliferation of endothelial cells as well as enhances the expression of molecules related to angiogenesis like MMP-2, 9, VEGF, and TGF-β [46]. Additionally, miRNA-101 is downregulated in GBM as a result of that Enhancer of zeste homolog 2 (EZH2)-induced proliferation, migration, and angiogenesis. Inhibition of EZH2 in glioma reduced angiogenesis and tumor growth [47].

Several miRNAs have been identified to play a crucial role in angiogenesis, and the transfer of RNAs from GBM cells to brain endothelial cells through extracellular vesicles induces angiogenesis. miRNA-148a and miRNA-9-5p both are linked with glioma angiogenesis and poor patient survival. When miRNA-9 is supplied to human umbilical ECs (HUVEC) through GBM-derived EVs, the number and length of tubules that develop as a consequence are inextricably linked with miRNA-9 expression in HUVECs [48, 49]. Transcriptional study identified RGS5, SOX7, and ABCB1 as a miRNA-9 target. Out of these, RGS5 and SOX7 are crucial for angiogenesis and cellular proliferation [48, 50, 51]. In experimental models of GBM, suppressing miRNA-148a normalizes the abnormal tumor angiogenesis [52].

Similarly, GSCs-derived miRNA-26a promotes proliferation, migration, and angiogenesis through inhibition of PTEN [53]. Vascular endothelial growth factor (VEGF) and VEGF receptor transcriptional activity may be controlled by the transcription factor Myc-associated zinc finger protein (MAZ). MAZ expression is regulated through miRNA-125; consequently, miR-125b overexpression prevents tumor angiogenesis [54, 55]. Several other miRNAs are also identified such as miRNA-124-3p, miRNA-15b, and miRNA-152 that play important roles in glioma cell invasion and angiogenesis.

Neuropilin-1 (NRP-1) promotes GBM cell development and growth that suppress miRNA-124-3p expression [56], while miRNA-15b and miRNA-152 inhibit glioma cell migration and angiogenesis through NRP-2 and MMP-3, respectively [57].

3.3 MicroRNAs in the generation of glioma stem cells

When compared to normal brain samples, GBM contains dysregulated levels of many miRNAs that play a crucial role in the generation of stem cell-like properties [26]. Loss of function assay of miRNA-663a induces proliferation, migration, invasion as well as stem cell-like properties in glioma. Gain of function assay shows overexpression of miRNA-663a represses cancer stem cell-like properties *via* inhibiting lysine demethylase 2A-mediated TGF-β/SMAD signaling pathway [58]. MiRNA-7 controls master regulators like the HoxD family of proteins as well as particular neuron activities including synaptic transmission. In line with its function in differentiation and proliferation, it has been identified as one of the miRNAs comprising the "miRNA signature" in neural stem and neural cancer stem cells [59]. The miRNA-9 is much more expressed in GBM CSF, GSCs, and GSC-derived EVs, which contributes to the aggressiveness of the disease; however, miRNA-9 inhibition had the opposite anticancer impact [60].

A microarray-based screening of 455 high-grade glioma patients identified differences in the level of miRNA-10a, miRNA-10b, and miRNA-139 that are crucial for the growth and differentiation of GSCs [61]. Enhanced differentiation of neurons was seen in murine astrocytic neural stem cells, murine oligodendroglioma-derived S100-v-erbB+ stem cells, human GBM CD133+ CSCs, and GBM cell lines after transfection with miRNA-124a or miRNA-137. In addition, G0/G1 cell cycle arrest and reduced expression of cell cycle components CDK6 and phosphorylated Rb were seen after co-transfection of miRNA-124a and miRNA-137 in GBM [62]. The miRNA-302-367 inhibits clonal development and SHH/GLI1/NANONG network regulation in GBM cells by targeting CXC chemokine receptor type 4 (CXCR4) and its ligand, stromal-derived factor 1 (SDF1). These findings suggest that miRNA-302-367 regulated a key pathway essential for the regeneration of neuron and stem cell phenotype [62]. Downregulation of miRNA-29b and miRNA-125a in CD133+ GSCs was also documented [63]. Similarly, like miRNA-125a, miRNA-125b plays a critical function in controlling the expansion of GBM cells and the activity of CSCs. A reduction in miRNA-125b in GBM cells was seen after all-trans-retinoic acid treatment [64].

Several other studies also identified miRNA dysregulation in GSCs compared to GBMs. Recent studies found miRNA-128a-3p, 34-5p, and 181a-3p to be downregulated, whereas miRNA-17-5p and miRNA-221-3p were increased in stem-like cells [65]. Also, miRNA-145 was typically under-expressed in GCSs, and its upregulation enhances chemosensitivity and cellular apoptosis [66]. MiRNA-27a-3p, miRNA-22-3p, and miRNA-221-3p were delivered to GSCs by EVs from monocyte-derived macrophages, and by concurrently targeting CHD7. These miRNAs induced proneural-to-mesenchymal transition in GSCs [67]. The miRNA expression profile reveals MiR-9, miR-9(*), miR-17, and miR-106b to be significantly abundant in CD133(+) cells, which also include populations of GSCs [68].

3.4 MicroRNAs in drug resistance in glioma

Several mechanisms of drug resistance include dysfunctional DNA repair, overexpression of drug efflux transporters, apoptosis inhibition, and increased epithelial-to-mesenchymal transition. The expression levels of MDR transporters are significantly impacted by miRNAs, which play a crucial role in controlling glioblastoma MDR [69]. Among the ABC transporter family, ABCG2 is particularly prominent in glioblastoma [70]. Downregulation of miRNA-328 reduces ABCG2 expression and chemoresistance in glioblastoma, suggesting that miRNA-328 plays a critical role in ABCG2 expression [71]. Therefore, miR-328 therapy combined with radiation or chemotherapy may be a useful approach for treating GBM [72]. Likewise, miRNA-1268a is downregulated after the TMZ treatment as a result of its target membrane transporter ABCC1/MRP1 being upregulated. Contrarily, overexpression of miRNA-1238a inhibits protein translation of ABCC1 and restores sensitivity to Temozolomide (TMZ) [73]. Moreover, by repressing miR-128-3p's effects on MRP1, RUNX1 makes GBM resistant to TMZ. Overcoming TMZ resistance in GBM may be possible *via* targeting the miR-128-3p/RUNX1/MRP1 axis [74].

Reversal of MDR in glioblastoma cells is also described after overexpression of miR-9 levels, which is associated with the suppression of ABC transporters such as MDR1, ABCC3, and ABCC6 [75]. In GBM, miRNA-381 was shown to be overexpressed; blocking miRNA-381 or driving neurofilament light polypeptide (NEFL) expression and greatly sensitizing GBM cells to the chemotherapeutic drug TMZ. Multiple multidrug resistance proteins (ABCG2, ABCC3, and ABCC5) and stemness factors (ALDH1, CD44, CKIT, KLF4, Nanog, Nestin, and SOX2) are the possible target of miRNA-381 by which these cells are sensitized to TMZ [76]. The ABCB1 is another drug efflux transporter that is overexpressed in resistant GBM cells and the study identified that expression of the transporter is controlled through miRNA-4539 and miRNA-4261 [77]. The aforementioned research emphasizes the importance of miRNA in ABC transporter-mediated drug efflux and suggests it as a viable therapeutic target for reestablishing chemosensitivity in gliomas.

Temozolomide is a first-choice alkylating agent inducted as a standard therapy for GBM and astrocytoma [78]. TMZ has limited efficacy due to the development of intrinsic and extrinsic drug resistance [79]. TMZ is an alkylating agent that generates methyldiazonium cation transfers their methyl group on N7 and O6 sites of guanine and the N3 on adenine [80]. The TMZ adduct imparts mutation in DNA fixed *via* O6-methylguanine-DNA methyltransferase (MGMT), Mismatch Repair (MMR), and Base Excision Repair (BER). MMR generates DNA double-strand breaks (DSBs) in TMZ-sensitive cells and triggers PCD, whereas overexpression of MGMT and other repair proteins remove TMZ adducts and generate TMZ-resistant glioma cells [11].

DNA mismatch repair (MMR) is a mechanism that detects and repairs DNA replication and recombination errors, including insertions, deletions, and misincorporations of nucleotides [81]. Compared to other cell types, radioresistant glioma cells had considerably high levels of DNA2 and low levels of miR-3059-3p. It has been identified that miR-3059-3p regulates radioresistance by targeting DNA2 and controlling homologous recombination pathways through Rad51 & 52. MiR-3059-3p-mediated downregulation of DNA2 inhibited the HR pathway, making GBM cells more radiosensitive [82]. Glioma cell proliferation is inhibited and senescence-related genes p53, Cdkn1a, and Cdkn2c are upregulated after delivery of miR-34a. Increased levels of miR-34a also reduce telomerase activity, shorten telomeres, and cause DNA damage. Forced overexpression of SIRT1 can counteract these pro-senescent effects [83].

Patients with GBM exhibited downregulation of miRNA-198 [84]. Reduced levels of these miRNAs are associated with a worse outcome for patients. Increased chemosensitivity to TMZ is also associated with elevated expression of miRNA-198, as shown by *in vitro* and *in vivo* investigations. This was achieved by miRNA-198 inhibiting protein translation specifically of MGMT [85]. Likewise, the miRNA-370-3p, which is suppressed in GBM, when transfected into TMZ-resistant GBM cells, makes them more sensitive to the anticancer medication by reducing their ability to fix their genetic lesions. Studies suggest that MGMT is a direct target of miRNA-370-3p and this miRNA plays a crucial role in the restoration of chemoresistance in GBM [86].

Additionally, multiple studies have shown the role of miRNAs in GBM tumorigenesis and onset of chemoresistance via activation of base excision repair proteins such as PARP, XRCC, Rad51, and others [87]. miRNA-151a depletion led to the development of TMZ resistance. And according to another study, enhanced miRNA-151a production sensitizes TMZ-resistant GBM cells by decreasing XRCC4-mediated DNA repair [88].

4. MicroRNA as glioma diagnostic biomarker

As we discussed earlier, miRNAs act as either oncogenes or tumor suppressors in glioma. Changes in the expression of these molecules have been linked to several cancer types, making them a promising molecular tool for non-invasive cancer detection and prognosis [89]. Hereby, we list some of the miRNAs that could be of diagnostic and prognostic significance (**Table 1**).

S.No.	Name of miRNAs	Sample Type	Marker Type	Reference
1.	miRNA-21.	Tissue, Plasma, EVs, CSF, plasma, and serum.	Diagnostic and Prognostic.	[90–93]
2.	miRNA-128, miRNA-342-3p.	Plasma	Diagnostic and Prognostic.	[93]
3.	miRNA-221	Tissue, CSF, Plasma, and serum.	Diagnostic	[90, 94, 95]
4.	miRNA-451	EVs	Diagnostic	[96]
5.	miRNA-182	Tissue and Plasma.	Diagnostic	[97, 98]
6.	miRNA-27a	Tissue, EVs, and CSF.	Prognostic	[99, 100]
7.	miRNA-21-5p, miRNA-218-5p, miRNA-193b-3p, miRNA-331-3p, miRNA-374a-5p, miRNA-548c-3p, miRNA-520f-3p, miRNA-27b-3p, miRNA-30b-3p.	CSF	Diagnostic, Prognostic.	[101]
8.	miRNA-125, miRNA-222.	CSF, Blood.	Diagnostic	[102]
9.	miRNA-10b	Tissue, CSF, Serum.	Diagnostic, Prognostic.	[92, 103]
10.	miRNA-183	Tissue	Prognostic	[104]

Table 1.
MiRNAs as a potential diagnostic and prognostic biomarker in glioma.

5. Therapeutic potential of miRNAs in glioma

Overall, the findings described in this chapter show that miRNAs are implicated in many pathways that worsen glioma patients' prognoses by promoting tumor growth, invasion, and resistance to therapy. What needs to be examined are the translational implications of these results and strategies to utilize this information in clinical practice. As we are aware, cancer is a complex disease that develops and spreads *via* the involvement of a variety of oncogenes and signaling mechanisms. The capacity of miRNA to concurrently target several genes involved in the same biochemical process is one of the numerous potential advantages of miRNA as a therapeutic agent. The two therapeutic focuses of miRNA-based treatment are miRNA replacement or antisense therapy and modulation of miRNA biogenesis [105]. DNA methylation and histone modification are two examples of epigenetic modulation that regulate certain miRNA biogenesis in cancer cells. Tumor-suppressing miRNAs can be activated with chromatin-modifying medications to control target oncogenes, which could pave the way to new cancer treatments in the near future [106]. A further advantage of miRNA mimics or replacement therapy is that they are predicted to target the same group of mRNAs that are controlled by the reduced original miRNA since they share the same sequence. Due to the designed imitation of miRNA mimics to replicate the behavior of their natural counterparts, the likelihood of experiencing any unintended off-target consequences is extremely low [107].

Scientists are actively investigating how to alter synthetic miRNAs to facilitate better translocation to host cells *in vivo* to increase the effectiveness of miRNAs in the field of cancer therapies. Several methods, including viral and non-viral alterations and chemical ones, are proposed to improve target delivery. For example, it is less probable for synthetic miRNAs to be degraded by nucleases if specific structural components, such as the 2'-OH of ribose or the phosphate backbone, are changed [108]. The cellular miRNAs' processing capacity is often poor and they are vulnerable to nuclease degradation, which reduces their bioavailability.

Recent studies also employ polymer nanoparticles as delivery vehicles for microRNAs (miRNAs) in GBM. Commonly used polymers include Poly (lactic-co-glycolic acid) or PLGA and Polyethyleneimine (PEI). Increased TMZ chemosensitivity was seen in both *in vitro* and *in vivo* after the delivery of antimiR-21 and antimiR-10b into GBM cells using PLGA nanoparticles [109–111]. Protecting miRNAs against degradation in a physiological environment is greatly aided by lipid nanoparticle delivery methods. Lipid nanoparticles are advantageous for transporting miRNAs in the clinic because of this quality. Complexes are readily formed when positively charged lipids are combined with negatively charged miRNAs through electrostatic interactions. These complexes increase the absorption rates of miRNAs [5, 112]. It is anticipated that if the delivery barrier is broken down and gaining a deeper knowledge of the effect and longevity of gene silencing, miRNAs are predicted to become useful therapies in the clinic.

6. Conclusion

Genome-wide profiling shows that miRNA expression is linked to tumor subtype, tumor grade, and patient outcomes in different cancers including glioma. Hence, miRNAs can be used as diagnostic, prognostic, and therapeutic biomarkers. Since it has been shown that miRNA deletion or overexpression is associated with glioma, researchers all over the globe have been trying to determine what functions miRNA play in cancer and what causes their expression to be dysregulated. MicroRNAs are hypothesized to behave as oncogenes or tumor suppressors in glioma by modifying particular targets. Numerous therapeutically promising miRNA antagonists and miRNA analogs are now in clinical trials, but further work is required to verify them as diagnostic and prognostic biomarkers in a large cohort of patient samples.

Acknowledgements

Manendra Singh Tomar is the recipient of a Junior research fellowship from the University Grants Commission, Government of India.

Declaration of interest

Authors declare no conflict of interest.

Author details

Manendra Singh Tomar and Ashutosh Shrivastava*
Faculty of Medicine, Center for Advance Research, King George's Medical University, Lucknow, Uttar Pradesh, India

*Address all correspondence to: ashutoshshrivastava@kgmcindia.edu

References

[1] Weller M, Wick W, Aldape K, Brada M, Berger M, Pfister SM, et al. Glioma. Nature Reviews. Disease Primers. 2015;**1**:15017. DOI: 10.1038/nrdp.2015.17

[2] Tomar MS, Shrivastava A. TERT promoter mutations correlate with IDHs, MGMT and EGFR in glioblastoma Multiforme. Neurology India. 2021;**69**(1):135-136. DOI: 10.4103/0028-3886.310071

[3] Brito C, Azevedo A, Esteves S, Marques AR, Martins C, Costa I, et al. Clinical insights gained by refining the 2016 WHO classification of diffuse gliomas with: EGFR amplification, TERT mutations, PTEN deletion and MGMT methylation. BMC Cancer. 2019;**19**(1):968. DOI: 10.1186/s12885-019-6177-0

[4] Hanif F, Muzaffar K, Perveen K, Malhi SM, Simjee Sh U. Glioblastoma Multiforme: A review of its epidemiology and pathogenesis through clinical presentation and treatment. Asian Pacific Journal of Cancer Prevention. 2017;**18**(1):3-9. DOI: 10.22034/apjcp.2017.18.1.3

[5] Chen M, Medarova Z, Moore A. Role of microRNAs in glioblastoma. Oncotarget. 2021;**12**(17):1707-1723. DOI: 10.18632/oncotarget.28039

[6] Lee SY. Temozolomide resistance in glioblastoma multiforme. Genes & Diseases. 2016;**3**(3):198-210. DOI: 10.1016/j.gendis.2016.04.007

[7] Bartel DP. Metazoan MicroRNAs. Cell. 2018;**173**(1):20-51. DOI: 10.1016/j.cell.2018.03.006

[8] Macfarlane LA, Murphy PR. MicroRNA: Biogenesis, function and role in cancer. Current Genomics. 2010;**11**(7):537-561. DOI: 10.2174/138920210793175895

[9] Calin GA, Sevignani C, Dumitru CD, Hyslop T, Noch E, Yendamuri S, et al. Human microRNA genes are frequently located at fragile sites and genomic regions involved in cancers. Proceedings of the National Academy of Sciences of the United States of America. 2004;**101**(9):2999-3004. DOI: 10.1073/pnas.0307323101

[10] Banelli B, Forlani A, Allemanni G, Morabito A, Pistillo MP, Romani M. MicroRNA in glioblastoma: An overview. International Journal of Genomics. 2017;**2017**:7639084. DOI: 10.1155/2017/7639084

[11] Tomar MS, Kumar A, Srivastava C, Shrivastava A. Elucidating the mechanisms of Temozolomide resistance in gliomas and the strategies to overcome the resistance. Biochimica Et Biophysica Acta. Reviews on Cancer. 2021;**1876**(2):188616. DOI: 10.1016/j.bbcan.2021.188616

[12] Cheray M, Etcheverry A, Jacques C, Pacaud R, Bougras-Cartron G, Aubry M, et al. Cytosine methylation of mature microRNAs inhibits their functions and is associated with poor prognosis in glioblastoma multiforme. Molecular Cancer. 2020;**19**(1):36. DOI: 10.1186/s12943-020-01155-z

[13] Miyoshi K, Miyoshi T, Siomi H. Many ways to generate microRNA-like small RNAs: Non-canonical pathways for microRNA production. Molecular Genetics and Genomics. 2010;**284**(2):95-103. DOI: 10.1007/s00438-010-0556-1

[14] Denli AM, Tops BB, Plasterk RH, Ketting RF, Hannon GJ. Processing

of primary microRNAs by the microprocessor complex. Nature. 2004;**432**(7014):231-235. DOI: 10.1038/nature03049

[15] Alarcón CR, Lee H, Goodarzi H, Halberg N, Tavazoie SF. N6-methyladenosine marks primary microRNAs for processing. Nature. 2015;**519**(7544):482-485. DOI: 10.1038/nature14281

[16] Lee D, Shin C. Emerging roles of DROSHA beyond primary microRNA processing. RNA Biology. 2018;**15**(2):186-193. DOI: 10.1080/15476286.2017.1405210

[17] Wu K, He J, Pu W, Peng Y. The role of Exportin-5 in MicroRNA biogenesis and cancer. Genomics, Proteomics & Bioinformatics. 2018;**16**(2):120-126. DOI: 10.1016/j.gpb.2017.09.004

[18] Medley JC, Panzade G, Zinovyeva AY. microRNA strand selection: Unwinding the rules. Wiley Interdisciplinary Reviews RNA. 2021;**12**(3):e1627. DOI: 10.1002/wrna.1627

[19] Zhang Y. RNA-induced silencing complex (RISC). In: Dubitzky W, Wolkenhauer O, Cho K-H, Yokota H, editors. Encyclopedia of Systems Biology. New York, New York, NY: Springer; 2013. DOI: 10.1007/978-1-4419-9863-7_329

[20] O'Brien J, Hayder H, Zayed Y, Peng C. Overview of MicroRNA biogenesis, mechanisms of actions, and circulation. Frontiers in Endocrinology (Lausanne). 2018;**9**:402. DOI: 10.3389/fendo.2018.00402

[21] Tarallo R, Giurato G, Bruno G, Ravo M, Rizzo F, Salvati A, et al. The nuclear receptor ERβ engages AGO2 in regulation of gene transcription, RNA splicing and RISC loading. Genome Biology. 2017;**18**(1):189. DOI: 10.1186/s13059-017-1321-0

[22] Ruby JG, Jan CH, Bartel DP. Intronic microRNA precursors that bypass Drosha processing. Nature. 2007;**448**(7149):83-86. DOI: 10.1038/nature05983

[23] Lam JK, Chow MY, Zhang Y, Leung SW. siRNA versus miRNA as therapeutics for gene silencing. Molecular Therapy Nucleic Acids. 2015;**4**(9):e252. DOI: 10.1038/mtna.2015.23

[24] Mafi A, Rahmati A, Babaei Aghdam Z, Salami R, Salami M, Vakili O, et al. Recent insights into the microRNA-dependent modulation of gliomas from pathogenesis to diagnosis and treatment. Cellular & Molecular Biology Letters. 2022;**27**(1):65. DOI: 10.1186/s11658-022-00354-4

[25] Srinivasan S, Patric IR, Somasundaram K. A ten-microRNA expression signature predicts survival in glioblastoma. PLoS One. 2011;**6**(3):e17438. DOI: 10.1371/journal.pone.0017438

[26] Møller HG, Rasmussen AP, Andersen HH, Johnsen KB, Henriksen M, Duroux M. A systematic review of microRNA in glioblastoma multiforme: Micro-modulators in the mesenchymal mode of migration and invasion. Molecular Neurobiology. 2013;**47**(1):131-144. DOI: 10.1007/s12035-012-8349-7

[27] Aloizou AM, Pateraki G, Siokas V, Mentis AA, Liampas I, Lazopoulos G, et al. The role of MiRNA-21 in gliomas: Hope for a novel therapeutic intervention? Toxicology Reports. 2020;7:1514-1530. DOI: 10.1016/j.toxrep.2020.11.001

[28] Yeh M, Wang YY, Yoo JY, Oh C, Otani Y, Kang JM, et al. MicroRNA-138 suppresses glioblastoma proliferation through downregulation of CD44. Scientific Reports. 2021;**11**(1):9219. DOI: 10.1038/s41598-021-88615-8

[29] Figueroa J, Phillips LM, Shahar T, Hossain A, Gumin J, Kim H, et al. Exosomes from glioma-associated mesenchymal stem cells increase the Tumorigenicity of glioma stem-like cells via transfer of miR-1587. Cancer Research. 2017;**77**(21):5808-5819. DOI: 10.1158/0008-5472.can-16-2524

[30] Buruiană A, Florian IȘ, Florian AI, Timiș TL, Mihu CM, Miclăuș M, et al. The roles of miRNA in glioblastoma tumor cell communication: Diplomatic and aggressive negotiations. International Journal of Molecular Sciences. 2020;**21**(6):1950. DOI: 10.3390/ijms21061950

[31] Huse JT, Brennan C, Hambardzumyan D, Wee B, Pena J, Rouhanifard SH, et al. The PTEN-regulating microRNA miR-26a is amplified in high-grade glioma and facilitates gliomagenesis in vivo. Genes & Development. 2009;**23**(11):1327-1337. DOI: 10.1101/gad.1777409

[32] Lu F, Li C, Sun Y, Jia T, Li N, Li H. Upregulation of miR-1825 inhibits the progression of glioblastoma by suppressing CDK14 though Wnt/β-catenin signaling pathway. World Journal of Surgical Oncology. 2020;**18**(1):147. DOI: 10.1186/s12957-020-01927-3

[33] Yan Y, Yan H, Wang Q, Zhang L, Liu Y, Yu H. MicroRNA 10a induces glioma tumorigenesis by targeting myotubularin-related protein 3 and regulating the Wnt/β-catenin signaling pathway. The FEBS Journal. 2019;**286**(13):2577-2592. DOI: 10.1111/febs.14824

[34] Wang J, Chen C, Yan X, Wang P. The role of miR-382-5p in glioma cell proliferation, migration and invasion. Oncotargets and Therapy. 2019;**12**:4993-5002. DOI: 10.2147/ott.s196322

[35] Wang Q, Li X, Zhu Y, Yang P. MicroRNA-16 suppresses epithelial-mesenchymal transition-related gene expression in human glioma. Molecular Medicine Reports. 2014;**10**(6):3310-3314. DOI: 10.3892/mmr.2014.2583

[36] Hagemann C, Anacker J, Ernestus RI, Vince GH. A complete compilation of matrix metalloproteinase expression in human malignant gliomas. World Journal of Clinical Oncology. 2012;**3**(5):67-79. DOI: 10.5306/wjco.v3.i5.67

[37] Wang X, Chen X, Sun L, Bi X, He H, Chen L, et al. MicroRNA-34a inhibits cell growth and migration in human glioma cells via MMP-9. Molecular Medicine Reports. 2019;**20**(1):57-64. DOI: 10.3892/mmr.2019.10233

[38] Peng G, Liu Y, Yang C, Shen C. MicroRNA-25 promotes cell proliferation, migration and invasion in glioma by directly targeting cell adhesion molecule 2. Experimental and Therapeutic Medicine. 2022;**23**(1):16. DOI: 10.3892/etm.2021.10938

[39] Li Y, Wang Y, Yu L, Sun C, Cheng D, Yu S, et al. miR-146b-5p inhibits glioma migration and invasion by targeting MMP16. Cancer Letters. 2013;**339**(2):260-269. DOI: 10.1016/j.canlet.2013.06.018

[40] Han J, Alvarez-Breckenridge CA, Wang QE, Yu J. TGF-β signaling and its targeting for glioma treatment. American Journal of Cancer Research. 2015;**5**(3):945-955

[41] Wang ZH, Zhang QS, Duan YL, Zhang JL, Li GF, Zheng DL. TGF-β induced miR-132 enhances the activation of TGF-β signaling through inhibiting SMAD7 expression in glioma cells. Biochemical and Biophysical Research Communications. 2015;**463**(3):187-192. DOI: 10.1016/j.bbrc.2015.05.001

[42] Li H, Li J, Chen L, Qi S, Yu S, Weng Z, et al. HERC3-mediated SMAD7

ubiquitination degradation promotes autophagy-induced EMT and Chemoresistance in glioblastoma. Clinical Cancer Research. 2019;**25**(12):3602-3616. DOI: 10.1158/1078-0432.ccr-18-3791

[43] Rosińska S, Gavard J. Tumor vessels fuel the fire in glioblastoma. International Journal of Molecular Sciences. 2021;**22**(12):6514. DOI: 10.3390/ijms22126514

[44] Ahir BK, Engelhard HH, Lakka SS. Tumor development and angiogenesis in adult brain tumor: Glioblastoma. Molecular Neurobiology. 2020;**57**(5):2461-2478. DOI: 10.1007/s12035-020-01892-8

[45] Würdinger T, Tannous BA, Saydam O, Skog J, Grau S, Soutschek J, et al. miR-296 regulates growth factor receptor overexpression in angiogenic endothelial cells. Cancer Cell. 2008;**14**(5):382-393. DOI: 10.1016/j.ccr.2008.10.005

[46] Dai D, Huang W, Lu Q, Chen H, Liu J, Hong B. miR-24 regulates angiogenesis in gliomas. Molecular Medicine Reports. 2018;**18**(1):358-368. DOI: 10.3892/mmr.2018.8978

[47] Smits M, Nilsson J, Mir SE, van der Stoop PM, Hulleman E, Niers JM, et al. Würdinger: miR-101 is down-regulated in glioblastoma resulting in EZH2-induced proliferation, migration, and angiogenesis. Oncotarget. 2010;**1**(8):710-720. DOI: 10.18632/oncotarget.205

[48] Chen X, Yang F, Zhang T, Wang W, Xi W, Li Y, et al. MiR-9 promotes tumorigenesis and angiogenesis and is activated by MYC and OCT4 in human glioma. Journal of Experimental & Clinical Cancer Research. 2019;**38**(1):99. DOI: 10.1186/s13046-019-1078-2

[49] Lucero R, Zappulli V, Sammarco A, Murillo OD, Cheah PS, Srinivasan S, et al. Glioma-derived miRNA-containing extracellular vesicles induce angiogenesis by reprogramming brain endothelial cells. Cell Reports. 2020;**30**(7):2065-2074.e4. DOI: 10.1016/j.celrep.2020.01.073

[50] Svensson A, Özen I, Genové G, Paul G, Bengzon J. Endogenous brain pericytes are widely activated and contribute to mouse glioma microvasculature. PLoS One. 2015;**10**(4):e0123553. DOI: 10.1371/journal.pone.0123553

[51] Kim K, Kim IK, Yang JM, Lee E, Koh BI, Song S, et al. SoxF transcription factors are positive feedback regulators of VEGF signaling. Circulation Research. 2016;**119**(7):839-852. DOI: 10.1161/circresaha.116.308483

[52] Wong HA, Fatimy RE, Onodera C, Wei Z, Yi M, Mohan A, et al. The cancer genome atlas analysis predicts MicroRNA for targeting cancer growth and vascularization in glioblastoma. Molecular Therapy. 2015;**23**(7):1234-1247. DOI: 10.1038/mt.2015.72

[53] Wang ZF, Liao F, Wu H, Dai J. Glioma stem cells-derived exosomal miR-26a promotes angiogenesis of microvessel endothelial cells in glioma. Journal of Experimental & Clinical Cancer Research. 2019;**38**(1):201. DOI: 10.1186/s13046-019-1181-4

[54] Yuan M, Da Silva A, Arnold A, Okeke L, Ames H, Correa-Cerro LS, et al. MicroRNA (miR) 125b regulates cell growth and invasion in pediatric low grade glioma. Scientific Reports. 2018;**8**(1):12506. DOI: 10.1038/s41598-018-30942-4

[55] Smits M, Wurdinger T, van het Hof B, Drexhage JA, Geerts D, Wesseling P, et al. Myc-associated zinc

finger protein (MAZ) is regulated by miR-125b and mediates VEGF-induced angiogenesis in glioblastoma. The FASEB Journal. 2012;**26**(6):2639-2647. DOI: 10.1096/fj.11-202820

[56] Zhang G, Chen L, Khan AA, Li B, Gu B, Lin F, et al. miRNA-124-3p/neuropilin-1(NRP-1) axis plays an important role in mediating glioblastoma growth and angiogenesis. International Journal of Cancer. 2018;**143**(3):635-644. DOI: 10.1002/ijc.31329

[57] Zheng X, Chopp M, Lu Y, Buller B, Jiang F. MiR-15b and miR-152 reduce glioma cell invasion and angiogenesis via NRP-2 and MMP-3. Cancer Letters. 2013;**329**(2):146-154. DOI: 10.1016/j.canlet.2012.10.026

[58] Wang L, Lang B, Zhou Y, Ma J, Hu K. Up-regulation of miR-663a inhibits the cancer stem cell-like properties of glioma via repressing the KDM2A-mediated TGF-β/SMAD signaling pathway. Cell Cycle. 2021;**20**(19):1935-1952. DOI: 10.1080/15384101.2021.1966962

[59] Korać P, Antica M, Matulić M. MiR-7 in cancer development. Biomedicine. 2021;**9**(3):325. DOI: 10.3390/biomedicines9030325

[60] Geng L, Xu J, Zhu Y, Hu X, Liu Y, Yang K, et al. Targeting miR-9 in glioma stem cell-derived extracellular vesicles: A novel diagnostic and therapeutic biomarker. Translational Oncology. 2022;**22**:101451. DOI: 10.1016/j.tranon.2022.101451

[61] Liu A, Zhao H, Sun B, Han X, Zhou D, Cui Z, et al. A predictive analysis approach for paediatric and adult high-grade glioma: miRNAs and network insight. The Annals of Translational Medicine. 2020;**8**(5):242. DOI: 10.21037/atm.2020.01.12

[62] Karsy M, Arslan E, Moy F. Current Progress on understanding MicroRNAs in glioblastoma Multiforme. Genes & Cancer. 2012;**3**(1):3-15. DOI: 10.1177/1947601912448068

[63] Cortez MA, Nicoloso MS, Shimizu M, Rossi S, Gopisetty G, Molina JR, et al. miR-29b and miR-125a regulate podoplanin and suppress invasion in glioblastoma. Genes, Chromosomes & Cancer. 2010;**49**(11):981-990. DOI: 10.1002/gcc.20808

[64] Xia HF, He TZ, Liu CM, Cui Y, Song PP, Jin XH, et al. MiR-125b expression affects the proliferation and apoptosis of human glioma cells by targeting Bmf. Cellular Physiology and Biochemistry. 2009;**23**(4-6):347-358. DOI: 10.1159/000218181

[65] Macharia LW, Muriithi W, Nyaga DK, de Mattos Coelho-Aguiar J. De Sampaio TCL. e Spohr and V Moura Neto: Evaluation of MiRNA expression in glioblastoma stem-like cells: A comparison between Normoxia and hypoxia microenvironment. Onco. 2022;**2**(2):113-128

[66] Qian C, Wang B, Zou Y, Zhang Y, Hu X, Sun W, et al. MicroRNA 145 enhances chemosensitivity of glioblastoma stem cells to demethoxycurcumin. Cancer Management and Research. 2019;**11**:6829-6840. DOI: 10.2147/cmar.s210076

[67] Zhang Z, Xu J, Chen Z, Wang H, Xue H, Yang C, et al. Transfer of MicroRNA via macrophage-derived extracellular vesicles promotes proneural-to-mesenchymal transition in glioma stem cells. Cancer Immunology Research. 2020;**8**(7):966-981. DOI: 10.1158/2326-6066.cir-19-0759

[68] Schraivogel D, Weinmann L, Beier D, Tabatabai G, Eichner A, Zhu JY, et al.

CAMTA1 is a novel tumour suppressor regulated by miR-9/9* in glioblastoma stem cells. The EMBO Journal. 2011;**30**(20):4309-4322. DOI: 10.1038/emboj.2011.301

[69] Mahinfar P, Mansoori B, Rostamzadeh D, Baradaran B, Cho WC, Mansoori B. The role of microRNAs in multidrug resistance of glioblastoma. Cancers (Basel). 2022;**14**(13):3217. DOI: 10.3390/cancers14133217

[70] Müller P, Abdel Gaber SA, Zimmermann W, Wittig R, Stepp H. ABCG2 influence on the efficiency of photodynamic therapy in glioblastoma cells. Journal of Photochemistry and Photobiology. B. 2020;**210**:111963. DOI: 10.1016/j.jphotobiol.2020.111963

[71] Li WQ, Li YM, Tao BB, Lu YC, Hu GH, Liu HM, et al. Yu: Downregulation of ABCG2 expression in glioblastoma cancer stem cells with miRNA-328 may decrease their chemoresistance. Medical Science Monitor. 2010;**16**(10):Hy27-30

[72] Wu Z, Sun L, Wang H, Yao J, Jiang C, Xu W, et al. MiR-328 expression is decreased in high-grade gliomas and is associated with worse survival in primary glioblastoma. PLoS One. 2012;7(10):e47270. DOI: 10.1371/journal.pone.0047270

[73] Li Y, Liu Y, Ren J, Deng S, Yi G, Guo M, et al. miR-1268a regulates ABCC1 expression to mediate temozolomide resistance in glioblastoma. Journal of Neuro-Oncology. 2018;**138**(3):499-508. DOI: 10.1007/s11060-018-2835-3

[74] Xu J, Song J, Xiao M, Wang C, Zhang Q, Yuan X, et al. RUNX1 (RUNX family transcription factor 1), a target of microRNA miR-128-3p, promotes temozolomide resistance in glioblastoma multiform by upregulating multidrug resistance-associated protein 1 (MRP1). Bioengineered. 2021;**12**(2):11768-11781. DOI: 10.1080/21655979.2021.2009976

[75] Jeon HM, Sohn YW, Oh SY, Kim SH, Beck S, Kim S, et al. ID4 imparts chemoresistance and cancer stemness to glioma cells by derepressing miR-9*-mediated suppression of SOX2. Cancer Research. 2011;**71**(9):3410-3421. DOI: 10.1158/0008-5472.can-10-3340

[76] Wang Z, Yang J, Xu G, Wang W, Liu C, Yang H, et al. Targeting miR-381-NEFL axis sensitizes glioblastoma cells to temozolomide by regulating stemness factors and multidrug resistance factors. Oncotarget. 2015;**6**(5):3147-3164. DOI: 10.18632/oncotarget.3061

[77] Medarova Z, Pantazopoulos P, Yoo B. Screening of potential miRNA therapeutics for the prevention of multi-drug resistance in cancer cells. Scientific Reports. 2020;**10**(1):1970. DOI: 10.1038/s41598-020-58919-2

[78] Strobel H, Baisch T, Fitzel R, Schilberg K, Siegelin MD, Karpel-Massler G, et al. Temozolomide and other alkylating agents in glioblastoma therapy. Biomedicine. 2019;7(3):69. DOI: 10.3390/biomedicines7030069

[79] Hu Z, Mi Y, Qian H, Guo N, Yan A, Zhang Y, et al. A potential mechanism of Temozolomide resistance in glioma-Ferroptosis. Frontiers in Oncology. 2020;**10**:897. DOI: 10.3389/fonc.2020.00897

[80] Ortiz R, Perazzoli G, Cabeza L, Jiménez-Luna C, Luque R, Prados J, et al. Temozolomide: An updated overview of resistance mechanisms, nanotechnology advances and clinical applications. Current Neuropharmacology. 2021;**19**(4):513-537. DOI: 10.2174/1570159x18666200626204005

[81] Caccese M, Ius T, Simonelli M, Fassan M, Cesselli D, Dipasquale A, et al. Mismatch-repair protein expression in high-grade gliomas: A large retrospective multicenter study. International Journal of Molecular Sciences. 2020;**21**(18):6716. DOI: 10.3390/ijms21186716

[82] Cheng YW, Lin CJ, Kuo SH, Lieu AS, Chai CY, Tsai HP, et al. miR-3059-3p regulates glioblastoma Multiforme Radiosensitivity enhancement through the homologous recombination pathway of DNA repair. Journal of Oncology. 2022;**2022**:7250278. DOI: 10.1155/2022/7250278

[83] Li Q, Wang C, Cai L, Lu J, Zhu Z, Wang C, et al. miR-34a derived from mesenchymal stem cells stimulates senescence in glioma cells by inducing DNA damage. Molecular Medicine Reports. 2019;**19**(3):1849-1857. DOI: 10.3892/mmr.2018.9800

[84] Yang L, Ma Y, Xin Y, Han R, Li R, Hao X. Role of the microRNA 181 family in glioma development. Molecular Medicine Reports. 2018;**17**(1):322-329. DOI: 10.3892/mmr.2017.7895

[85] Nie E, Jin X, Wu W, Yu T, Zhou X, Shi Z, et al. MiR-198 enhances temozolomide sensitivity in glioblastoma by targeting MGMT. Journal of Neuro-Oncology. 2017;**133**(1):59-68. DOI: 10.1007/s11060-017-2425-9

[86] Gao YT, Chen XB, Liu HL. Up-regulation of miR-370-3p restores glioblastoma multiforme sensitivity to temozolomide by influencing MGMT expression. Scientific Reports. 2016;**6**:32972. DOI: 10.1038/srep32972

[87] Bandey I, Chiou SH, Huang AP, Tsai JC, Tu PH. Progranulin promotes Temozolomide resistance of glioblastoma by orchestrating DNA repair and tumor stemness. Oncogene. 2015;**34**(14):1853-1864. DOI: 10.1038/onc.2014.92

[88] Zeng A, Wei Z, Yan W, Yin J, Huang X, Zhou X, et al. Exosomal transfer of miR-151a enhances chemosensitivity to temozolomide in drug-resistant glioblastoma. Cancer Letters. 2018;**436**:10-21. DOI: 10.1016/j.canlet.2018.08.004

[89] Filipów S, Łaczmański Ł. Blood circulating miRNAs as cancer biomarkers for diagnosis and surgical treatment response. Frontiers in Genetics. 2019;**10**:169. DOI: 10.3389/fgene.2019.00169

[90] Conti A, Aguennouz M, La Torre D, Tomasello C, Cardali S, Angileri FF, et al. miR-21 and 221 upregulation and miR-181b downregulation in human grade II-IV astrocytic tumors. Journal of Neuro-Oncology. 2009;**93**(3):325-332. DOI: 10.1007/s11060-009-9797-4

[91] Akers JC, Ramakrishnan V, Kim R, Phillips S, Kaimal V, Mao Y, et al. miRNA contents of cerebrospinal fluid extracellular vesicles in glioblastoma patients. Journal of Neuro-Oncology. 2015;**123**(2):205-216. DOI: 10.1007/s11060-015-1784-3

[92] Teplyuk NM, Mollenhauer B, Gabriely G, Giese A, Kim E, Smolsky M, et al. MicroRNAs in cerebrospinal fluid identify glioblastoma and metastatic brain cancers and reflect disease activity. Neuro-Oncology. 2012;**14**(6):689-700. DOI: 10.1093/neuonc/nos074

[93] Wang Q, Li P, Li A, Jiang W, Wang H, Wang J, et al. Plasma specific miRNAs as predictive biomarkers for diagnosis and prognosis of glioma. Journal of Experimental & Clinical Cancer Research. 2012;**31**(1):97. DOI: 10.1186/1756-9966-31-97

[94] Godlewski J, Krichevsky AM, Johnson MD, Chiocca EA, Bronisz A. Belonging to a network--microRNAs, extracellular vesicles, and the glioblastoma microenvironment. Neuro-Oncology. 2015;**17**(5):652-662. DOI: 10.1093/neuonc/nou292

[95] Dong L, Li Y, Han C, Wang X, She L, Zhang H. miRNA microarray reveals specific expression in the peripheral blood of glioblastoma patients. International Journal of Oncology. 2014;**45**(2):746-756. DOI: 10.3892/ijo.2014.2459

[96] van der Vos KE, Abels ER, Zhang X, Lai C, Carrizosa E, Oakley D, et al. Directly visualized glioblastoma-derived extracellular vesicles transfer RNA to microglia/macrophages in the brain. Neuro-Oncology. 2016;**18**(1):58-69. DOI: 10.1093/neuonc/nov244

[97] Li E, Zhang J, Yuan T, Ma B. MiR-143 suppresses osteogenic differentiation by targeting Osterix. Molecular and Cellular Biochemistry. 2014;**390**(1-2):69-74. DOI: 10.1007/s11010-013-1957-3

[98] Quirico L, Orso F. The power of microRNAs as diagnostic and prognostic biomarkers in liquid biopsies. Cancer Drug Resistance. 2020;**3**(2):117-139. DOI: 10.20517/cdr.2019.103

[99] Rivera-Díaz M, Miranda-Román MA, Soto D, Quintero-Aguilo M, Ortiz-Zuazaga H, Marcos-Martinez MJ, et al. MicroRNA-27a distinguishes glioblastoma multiforme from diffuse and anaplastic astrocytomas and has prognostic value. American Journal of Cancer Research. 2015;**5**(1):201-218

[100] Huang SW, Ali ND, Zhong L, Shi J. MicroRNAs as biomarkers for human glioblastoma: Progress and potential. Acta Pharmacologica Sinica. 2018;**39**(9):1405-1413. DOI: 10.1038/aps.2017.173

[101] Akers JC, Hua W, Li H, Ramakrishnan V, Yang Z, Quan K, et al. A cerebrospinal fluid microRNA signature as biomarker for glioblastoma. Oncotarget. 2017;**8**(40):68769-68779. DOI: 10.18632/oncotarget.18332

[102] Wang J, Che F, Zhang J. Cell-free microRNAs as non-invasive biomarkers in glioma: A diagnostic meta-analysis. The International Journal of Biological Markers. 2019;**34**(3):232-242. DOI: 10.1177/1724600819840033

[103] Kim TM, Huang W, Park R, Park PJ, Johnson MD. A developmental taxonomy of glioblastoma defined and maintained by MicroRNAs. Cancer Research. 2011;**71**(9):3387-3399. DOI: 10.1158/0008-5472.can-10-4117

[104] Ye Z, Zhang Z, Wu L, Liu C, Chen Q, Liu J, et al. Upregulation of miR-183 expression and its clinical significance in human brain glioma. Neurological Sciences. 2016;**37**(8):1341-1347. DOI: 10.1007/s10072-016-2599-5

[105] Arghiani N, Shah K. Modulating microRNAs in cancer: Next-generation therapies. Cancer Biology & Medicine. 2021;**19**(3):289-304. DOI: 10.20892/j.issn.2095-3941.2021.0294

[106] Cho WC. OncomiRs: The discovery and progress of microRNAs in cancers. Molecular Cancer. 2007;**6**:60. DOI: 10.1186/1476-4598-6-60

[107] Bader AG, Brown D, Winkler M. The promise of microRNA replacement therapy. Cancer Research. 2010;**70**(18):7027-7030. DOI: 10.1158/0008-5472.can-10-2010

[108] Bhat SA, Majid S, Rehman MU. Scenario and future prospects of microRNAs in gastric cancer: A review. Iranian Journal of Basic Medical Sciences. 2019;**22**(4):345-352. DOI: 10.22038/ijbms.2019.32399.7765

[109] Ananta JS, Paulmurugan R, Massoud TF. Nanoparticle-delivered antisense MicroRNA-21 enhances the effects of Temozolomide on glioblastoma cells. Molecular Pharmaceutics. 2015;**12**(12):4509-4517. DOI: 10.1021/acs.molpharmaceut.5b00694

[110] Ananta JS, Paulmurugan R, Massoud TF. Tailored nanoparticle Codelivery of antimiR-21 and antimiR-10b augments glioblastoma cell kill by Temozolomide: Toward a "personalized" anti-microRNA therapy. Molecular Pharmaceutics. 2016;**13**(9):3164-3175. DOI: 10.1021/acs.molpharmaceut.6b00388

[111] Malhotra M, Sekar TV, Ananta JS, Devulapally R, Afjei R, Babikir HA, et al. Targeted nanoparticle delivery of therapeutic antisense microRNAs presensitizes glioblastoma cells to lower effective doses of temozolomide in vitro and in a mouse model. Oncotarget. 2018;**9**(30):21478-21494. DOI: 10.18632/oncotarget.25135

[112] Chen Y, Gao DY, Huang L. In vivo delivery of miRNAs for cancer therapy: Challenges and strategies. Advanced Drug Delivery Reviews. 2015;**81**:128-141. DOI: 10.1016/j.addr.2014.05.009

Chapter 4

Magnetic Nanocarrier Based Drug Targeting: Emerging Trend for the Treatment of Glioma

Bhabani Sankar Satapathy, Jnanranjan Panda, Biswabhusan Biswal, Abhishek Mishra, Snigdha Pattnaik, Pralaya Kumar Sahoo and Anshuman Gouda

Abstract

Effective treatment of glioma; the most aggressive primary brain tumor has been a worrisome medical challenge across the globe. Owing to the architectural uniqueness of the brain coupled with the presence of the blood-brain barrier hijacks the success of conventional treatment strategies. In this context, magnetic nanocarriers (MNCs) have garnered significant attention over the past decade as efficient imaging and targeted drug delivery platforms in glioma. In many recent research, ferrite-based drug carriers have shown preferential anticancer activity against glioma cells both *in vitro* and *in vivo*. Under the influence of an externally applied magnetic field, anticancer drug-loaded MNCs could be directed at specific tumor locations and can release the cytotoxic drugs more precisely at the tumor area, thereby reducing off-target toxic effects. Among the ferrite-based MNCs, superparamagnetic nanocarriers are considered more biocompatible. Further, the outer surface of MNCs is coated with biodegradable hydrophilic polymers like PEG to make them suitable for in *vivo* applications. Additionally, MNCs can be functionalized with specific ligands like monoclonal antibodies, peptides, aptamers, etc., to improve tumor-specific targeting. The chapter highlights research advancements in MNCs-based drug targeting investigated over the past years for the treatment of glioma along with key challenges on the roads of technology transfer for industrial viability.

Keywords: magnetic nanocarriers, glioma, drug targeting, advancements, challenges

1. Introduction

Glioma is a type of brain tumor that originates in the glial cells, which are supportive cells of the central nervous system. Glial cells provide structural support, nourishment, and insulation to neurons. Gliomas are the most common type of primary brain tumor, accounting for approximately 80% of all malignant brain tumors, they originate within the brain or spinal cord, as opposed to spreading from other parts of the body [1]. Gliomas can occur in individuals of any age but are more

IntechOpen

frequently diagnosed in adults. The exact causes of gliomas are not well understood, although certain genetic and environmental factors may play a role [2]. Exposure to ionizing radiation, genetic predisposition, and some rare genetic disorders have been associated with an increased risk of developing gliomas. Gliomas can occur in people of all ages, but they are most commonly diagnosed in adults between the ages of 45 and 65 [3]. These tumors can be classified into different types based on the specific glial cell they originate from. The three main types of gliomas are astrocytoma, oligodendroglioma, and ependymoma. Astrocytomas are the most common type of glioma and arise from astrocytes, which are star-shaped glial cells. They are further categorized into grades I–IV based on their level of aggressiveness, with grade IV being the most malignant form, known as glioblastoma multiforme (GBM) [4]. Oligodendrogliomas originate from oligodendrocytes, which are responsible for producing myelin, a substance that insulates nerve fibers. These tumors are usually slow-growing and occur more commonly in adults. Ependymomas develop from ependymal cells that line the ventricles of the brain and the center of the spinal cord. They are more commonly found in children and young adults [5]. Treatment options for glioma depend on several factors, including the tumor grade, location, and overall health of the patient. The main treatments for glioma include surgery, radiation therapy, and chemotherapy. In some cases, a combination of these treatments may be used. The goal of treatment is to remove as much of the tumor as possible, slow down its growth, and manage symptoms to improve the patient's quality of life [6]. Symptoms of gliomas can vary depending on the size, location, and rate of growth of the tumor. Common symptoms may include headaches, seizures, cognitive and memory problems, changes in behavior or personality, difficulty with balance and coordination, and neurological deficits. The diagnosis of gliomas typically involves a combination of medical history evaluation, neurological examination, imaging tests such as MRI or CT scans, and sometimes a biopsy to confirm the presence of tumor cells [7].

Treatment of glioma, the most common form of brain tumor has been a tough challenge to treat and often necessitates novel targeting strategies [8]. Gliomas are highly aggressive and invasive, and their location in the brain makes them difficult to access and treat. The current standard treatments, including surgery, chemotherapy, and radiation therapy, have several limitations, such as low therapeutic efficacy, high toxicity, and drug resistance. Hence, there is an urgent need for novel and effective therapeutic strategies for glioma [9].

Nanotechnology has recently become a potential method for treating gliomas. Nanoparticles have unique physical and chemical properties that make them suitable for drug delivery applications. Among the various types of nanoparticles, magnetic nanocarriers have gained significant attention due to their ability to selectively target and deliver drugs to the tumor site, enhance drug accumulation, and reduce systemic toxicity [10].

Magnetic nanocarriers are composed of a magnetic core, which allows for magnetic targeting, and a shell, which can be functionalized with various ligands to improve tumor-specific accumulation. The magnetic core is typically composed of iron oxide, which is biocompatible and biodegradable [11]. The shell can be made of various materials, such as lipids, polymers, and silica, depending on the desired properties. One of the main advantages of magnetic nanocarriers is their ability to selectively target the tumor site using an external magnetic field. As a result, the loaded drug can be more precisely accumulated at the tumor site, while reducing systemic toxicity [12]. Additionally, magnetic nanocarriers can be functionalized with various ligands, such as antibodies, peptides, and aptamers, to improve tumor-specific targeting and reduce off-target effects. Another advantage of magnetic nanocarriers is their ability to overcome the blood-brain barrier (BBB), which is a major obstacle in the treatment of glioma [13]. The BBB is a complex structure of endothelial cells, which tightly regulates the passage of substances between the bloodstream and the brain. The BBB limits the penetration of most chemotherapeutic drugs into the brain, which hinders the efficacy of glioma treatment. However, magnetic nanocarriers can cross the BBB using magnetic targeting and can deliver drugs directly to the tumor site [14].

2. Blood-brain barrier

The blood-brain barrier (BBB) serves as a diffusion barrier that prevents poisons and other substances from entering the brain while safeguarding the brain's neuronal tissues. Two different types of cellular junctions, the paracellular tight junction and the intercellular adherens junction, are present in the BBB based on its molecular construction [15]. Adherens junction, which is made up of cadherin, vascular endothelium (VE), catenin, and actinin maintains the BBB's functional quality. Tight junctions, however, retain the BBB's primary functioning because they are principally in charge of permeability via the BBB. A complicated cellular network makes up the BBB in adults. Brain endothelial cells, a highly specialized basal membrane, many pericytes surrounding the basal membrane, and astrocytic end-feet were the primary elements of this system [16].

2.1 Brain endothelial cells

For effective barrier construction and interactions with neighboring cells, such cells are necessary. Also, they are referred as brain microvascular endothelial cells (BMECs). The following are some ways that BMECs are different from endothelial cells found in other organs: (i) Consistent tight connections among brain endothelial cells stop chemicals from moving across cells, (ii) BMECs contain more mitochondria and fewer cytoplasmic vesicles, & (iii) BMECs do not exhibit identifiable transendothelial pathways such as intracellular vesicular transport [17]. Complex intercellular tight junctions prevent chemicals from passively diffusing into the brain, which causes blood vessels to have exceptionally high transendothelial electrical resistance (TEER) in *vivo*. Additionally, BMECs have the capacity to transport molecules like efflux transporters (p-glycoprotein) across the BBB in addition to other necessary nutrients and metabolites. These transporters help the BBB's characteristics by allowing tiny lipophilic substances to escape into BMECs and then return to the blood stream [18].

2.2 Basal membrane

The whole surface of the capillary endothelial cell layers is covered by this structure, which is made up of type IV collagen, laminin, and fibronectin. This membrane has pericytes embedded inside it, and astrocytic end-feet surround them. This membrane's possible use is to prevent the solutes from moving around freely [19].

2.3 Pericytes

Pericytes are the contractile cells that surround the endothelial cells. These cells regulate the expression of BBB-specific genes in endothelial cells, induce polarization of astrocytic end-feet encircling CNS blood vessels, and prevent CNS immune cells from impairing the proper formation of BBB. Additionally, these cells assist in decreasing the expression of substances that raise vascular permeability [20].

2.4 Astrocytic end-feet

Previously, it was believed that the astrocytic end-feet surrounding endothelial cells did not significantly contribute to BBB maintenance [21]. On the other hand, recent research by Nuriya et al. (2013) revealed the variability of diffusion patterns surrounding astrocytic end-feet. They established the presence of certain astrocytic end-feet that can organize into compact networks and prevent molecules from diffusing freely through them. The variability of diffusion patterns is influenced by the different blood vessels & physical features of the gliovascular interface, such as the distance between endothelial cells & astrocytic end-feet. As a result, these networks firmly surround blood vessels, which raises the possibility that astrocytic end-feet serve functional purposes [22].

3. Molecular composition of BBB

The molecular composition of the BBB is complex and dynamic, and it is controlled by a number of variables, including the surrounding environment and the specific needs of the brain. Some of the key components of the BBB include:

a. *Tight junction proteins:* The endothelial cells that make up the BBB are connected by tight junctions, which form a barrier that prevents the free passage of molecules. Numerous proteins, such as claudins, occluding, and junctional adhesion molecules, are found in tight junctions [23].

b. *Transport proteins:* The BBB is highly selective in the molecules that allows to cross from the blood into the brain. This is achieved through the expression of specialized transport proteins that selectively move molecules across the endothelial cell layer. Examples of these transporters include glucose transporters, amino acid transporters, and efflux transporters that pump out potentially harmful substances [24].

c. *Enzymes:* The BBB also contains a variety of enzymes that regulate the transport and metabolism of molecules. For example, the enzyme monoamine oxidase helps to break down neurotransmitters like dopamine and serotonin [25].

d. *Adhesion molecules:* Adhesion molecules are proteins that help to maintain the structure and function of the BBB. These molecules include integrins and cadherins, which are important for cell-cell interactions and communication [26].

e. *Extracellular matrix components:* The extracellular matrix is a network of proteins and other molecules that provides structural support to cells. The BBB contains specific extracellular matrix components, such as laminin and collagen, which help to maintain the integrity of the endothelial cell layer [27].

f. Overall, the molecular composition of the BBB is highly specialized and tightly regulated, allowing for the selective transport of molecules between the blood and the brain while maintaining the overall health and function of the brain [28].

4. Targeting strategy of magnetic nanocarrier *vs.* conventional therapy

Nanocarriers are a promising approach for the treatment of glioma due to their ability to selectively target the tumor site, enhance drug accumulation, and reduce systemic toxicity [29]. In comparison, conventional therapies such as surgery, chemotherapy, and radiation therapy have several limitations, such as low therapeutic efficacy, high toxicity, and drug resistance. The targeting strategy of magnetic nanocarriers involves the use of an external magnetic field to guide the nanoparticles to the tumor site [30]. The magnetic field can be applied locally, allowing for precise targeting & increased drug accumulation at the tumor site, while reducing off-target effects. This targeted approach can also overcome the blood-brain barrier, which is a significant obstacle to the treatment of glioma, and deliver drugs directly to the tumor site [31].

In contrast, conventional therapies have limited tumor specificity, and a significant amount of the drug is distributed throughout the body, which results in systemic toxicity. Additionally, the blood-brain barrier limits the penetration of most chemotherapeutic drugs into the brain that blocks the efficacy of glioma treatment [32]. The strategy of drug targeting by MNCs in bypassing BBB in comparison to conventional drug therapy has been depicted in **Figure 1**. While surgery can remove a significant portion of the tumor, it is often not feasible for tumors located in critical brain regions. Moreover, conventional therapies often lead to drug resistance, limiting their long-term efficacy. Gliomas are highly heterogeneous, and the tumor cells can develop resistance to chemotherapy and radiation therapy, leading to treatment failure [33]. Magnetic nanocarriers can overcome drug resistance by delivering drugs directly to the tumor site, allowing for higher drug concentrations, and reducing the likelihood of drug resistance. In conclusion, magnetic nanocarriers offer several advantages over conventional

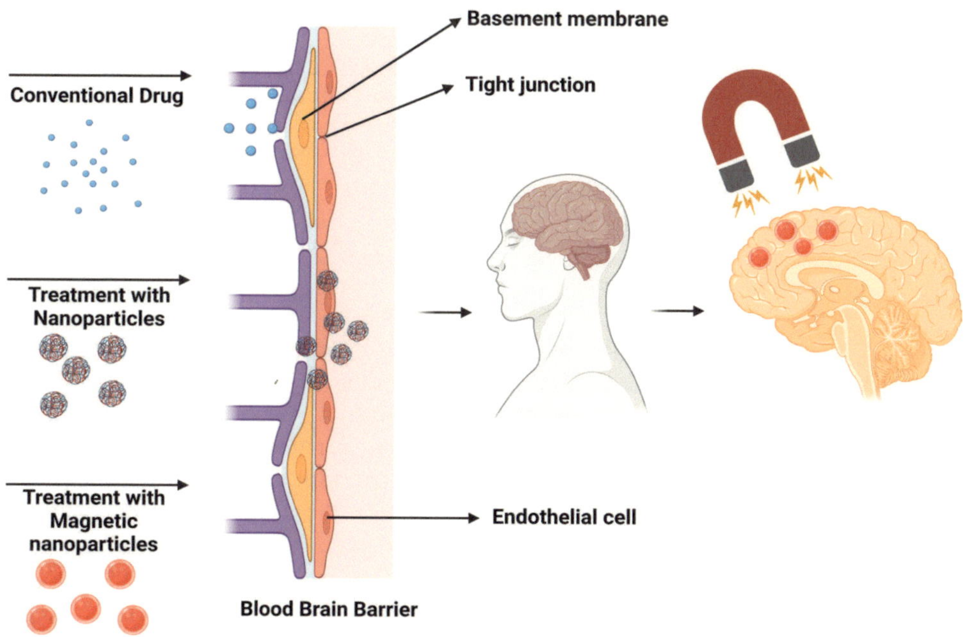

Figure 1.
Magnetic carrier vs. conventional drug therapy.

therapies for the treatment of glioma, including targeted drug delivery, enhanced drug accumulation, reduced systemic toxicity, and overcoming drug resistance. While there are still several challenges to overcome, including nanoparticle design optimization and magnetic targeting parameters, for the treatment of gliomas in the future, magnetic nanocarriers show enormous potential [34]. The effectiveness of magnetic nanocarriers over conventional therapy in tumor targeting has been summarized in **Figure 1**.

5. Types of magnetic nanocarrier

Magnetic nanocarriers are a type of nanoparticle that can be guided to specific cells or tissues using an external magnetic field. They have potential applications in a variety of fields, including drug delivery, imaging, and therapy. There are several types of magnetic nanocarriers, including:

a. *Iron oxide nanoparticles:* Iron oxide nanoparticles are among the most commonly used magnetic nanocarriers due to their biocompatibility and magnetic properties. They can be coated with various materials to improve their stability, targeting, and drug loading capacity [35].

b. *Magnetic liposomes:* Magnetic liposomes are liposomal structures that contain magnetic nanoparticles. They can be functionalized with various ligands to target specific cells or tissues and can be used for both diagnostic and therapeutic purposes [36].

c. *Magnetic polymeric nanoparticles:* Magnetic polymeric nanoparticles are polymeric structures that contain magnetic nanoparticles. They can be designed to be biodegradable, biocompatible, and capable of controlled drug release [37].

d. *Magnetic dendrimers:* Dendrimers are branched, synthetic molecules that can be functionalized with magnetic nanoparticles. They can be used for targeted drug delivery, imaging, and diagnostics [38].

6. Method of synthesis of MNCs

6.1 Physical methods

It consists of two processes like bottom-up & top-down. In the top-down process, larger particles were made into smaller ones. It is challenging to produce a uniform shape and size for an MNP via the mechanical method. In the bottom-up method, well dispersed ultra-micron size particles can be easily formed employing some physical processes like laser evaporation, inert gas condensation, etc. [39]. The processes are as follows,

6.1.1 Ball milling method/mechanical method

It helps to produce the MNCs in bulk amounts by a top-down approach. It is a process in which the grinding of coarse material into finer particles occurs. The basic operation involves placing raw materials in a jar with steel balls acting as a crushing component. Through the kinetic energy generated by balls, a collision occurs between the balls and the larger materials, which are crushed into smaller ones. The powder ball ratio, milling time, and vibration speed were chief controllers to form a nano-/micron-sized crystal. But due to the presence of iron balls and uncertain temperature inside the jar may causes some contamination to the materials [40].

6.1.2 Laser evaporation

It is processed exactly the opposite of the first method known as a bottom-up strategy where MNCs are prepared by condensation from a gaseous phase or liquid. It is also called laser ablation where the high-energy laser is applied. In this method, the coarse particles are evaporated under a laser beam, and the ingredients are positioned at the base of the liquid solution and passed through a laser beam. The irradiation occurs and when the vapor cools into a gaseous state, nucleation takes place which helps in the formation of MNCs. It is cheaper and does not require any high-cost chemicals, processes, and instruments [41].

6.1.3 Wire explosion method

It is a physiochemical technique that is a very effective and useful strategy to make the MNCs. Here no additional steps are required to separate out the NPs from a solution and again not involved in any processes to form by-products. It is a fully organized process and no contamination chances because it requires minimum energy [42].

6.2 Chemical methods

It processes through different bottom-up parts. Here are some comprehensive methods through which well-organized MNCs were formed by adding some newer technologies and some new ingredients.

6.2.1 Solution precipitation

In this process, a precipitating agent must be added to the meta precursor which creates a precipitate of insoluble materials and after precipitation it shows a high yield of products. The advantage is the uniformity of particles, nucleation, and growth of particles. Here the solution is prepared by taking $FeCl_3$ and NaOH solution at 50–100C. The solution is made more efficient by increasing temperature and by stirring process. Here the disadvantage is it requires a prolonged time to produce a complete solution followed by precipitation [43].

6.2.2 Co-precipitation method

Here magnetic nanoparticles are prepared in an aqueous solution of iron in anaerobic conditions at ambient temperature. Here some nanocrystals like Manganese ferrite ($MnFe_2O_4$) are prepared by using manganese chloride ($MnCl_2$) & ferric chloride ($FeCl_3$) as metal ions and salt of NaOH as a precipitant. From here nanocrystals are precipitated by the addition of NaOH which creates some metal ions at a certain temperature. But the main problem is to make it reproducible by allowing proper synthetic conditions. However, some ferrimagnetic materials by the process of oxidation adjust the pH, ionic strength, etc. [44].

6.2.3 Thermal decomposition approach

Here some organometallic precursors are immersed followed by surfactants are used under anaerobic zones as a capping agent for rotting in organic solvents which produces as MNCs. Fatty acids are employed as stabilizing agents in this instance to create MNCs. Which helps the material to be in a proper shape and size. Iron oxide MNCs must undergo oxidation in order to be formed; iron valent precursors $Fe(CO)_5$ are thermally decomposed to produce MNCs. To control the size, shape, and dispersion behavior they must possess it into some liquid organic material and vapor phases but in the presence of oxygen there must be some chemical reaction that creates challenges [45].

6.3 Polyol method

It is used in MNCs to synthesize uniform MNCs to show magnetic resonance imaging. These methods were water-compatible and chelation which processes to nuclei formation and helps to control the size, stability, and dispersibility of the product. Some polyols are PEG, TEG, Glycerol, etc. This part creates a layer on the MNCs to make it more shiner in texture having a proper size through which we can place it inside the brain and the magnetic field also accepts the material having a controlled release [46].

6.4 Microemulsion synthesis

It is prepared through thermodynamically stable isotropic preparation in the presence of interfacial layers of surfactant molecules, two identical micro emulsions are mixed then the appearance must be formed as a micelle by which the extraction is made through centrifugation. These are turbid emulsions having both hydrophilic and lipophilic phases and can be miscible with the help of surfactants and co-surfactants. This process is coordinated through two types i.e., O/W type, W/O type, supplied water & oil. It is also responsible for maintaining the shape and size of MNCs provided with the help of the effectiveness of the surfactants which is used. The majority of iron oxide MNCs are made using an emulsion of the W/O type and it's also known as nanoreactors to produce MNCs having some transition materials [47].

6.5 Hydrothermal method

It is also known as the solvothermal route to prepare MNCs and ultrafine powders, at different temperatures and different pressures. Here the main part to produce the MNCs are hydrolysis and oxidation. Due to the incorporation of an aqueous medium or water, the chances of crystal formation are dependent. The shape and crystallinity of MNCs are further explored through solvent mixing, time, temperature, and pressure quantity. This process needs high temperature and pressure. So, comparatively, it is preferred over the Sol-gel method for preparing proper shape, size, and high crystalline products. The challenge is the slowness of kinetic at certain temperatures which increases the rate of crystallization. If we use some reaction mixtures at a certain temperature and pressure, then the formation will be uniform [48].

6.6 Sol-Gel method

In this part, gel formation is needed first by hydrolysis and polycondensation at room temperature. Some metal salts are also used to prepare a sol solution and other colloidal solutions by dissolving in water or other solvents. The Vander Waals force is created in between the particles of the heated mixtures till all solvents are eliminated and the solution is dried completely. This method is very effective for the control of the composition of MNCs and somehow size and shape of MNCs. The mixture of $FeCl_3$ and NaOH is required at 50–100C. Sol-gel method does not require any instrument that's why it is very cheap method to prepare MNCs. But in some cases, it may cause some contamination from by-product reactions. The disadvantage is it may involve some toxic organic solvents [49].

6.7 Biological synthesis

It is processed through green chemistry by chemical manipulation which focuses on eliminating the toxic material from the environment. It starts with some micro-organisms & plants like algae, fungi, actinomycetes, & bacteria. The advantages of these methods are efficiency, eco-friendly, & an organized procedure; however, a drawback is the nanoparticles' poor dispersion. Particles having a size range of 60 nm ferromagnetic magnetite were ideal for biological synthesis. The mechanism of preparation of MNCs is the activity of nitrate reductase, mixed mechanism, and shuttle electrons quinones. But till now it is not very clear to prepare. So, Fe_3O_4 magnetic materials are used through a catalyst named photo-catalyst. Some metallic ingredients are carried through tissue, extract, and enzymes of living organisms to process a strong, nontoxic product [50].

7. Mechanism of magnetic nanocarrier for the treatment of glioma

The mechanism of magnetic nanocarriers for the treatment of glioma involves several steps, which are discussed below. Further, the overall mechanism of magnetic-oriented drug targeting at tumor cells has been depicted in **Figure 2**.

a. *Magnetic targeting*: Magnetic nanocarriers are guided to glioma cells using an external magnetic field. The magnetic field can be applied externally or implanted locally in the brain, allowing for precise targeting of the nanocarriers to the tumor site [51].

b. *Penetration across the BBB*: Once the magnetic nanocarriers are in proximity to the BBB, they can penetrate the endothelial cell layer and cross the BBB through several mechanisms. These may include passive diffusion, receptor-mediated transport, or transcytosis across the endothelial cells [52].

c. *Uptake by glioma cells*: Once the magnetic nanocarriers have crossed the BBB and reached the glioma cells, they can be taken up by the cells through various mechanisms, such as receptor-mediated endocytosis or phagocytosis [53].

d. *Controlled release of loaded cargo*: Magnetic nanocarriers can be designed to release their payload of drugs or other therapeutic agents in a controlled manner once they are inside the glioma cells. This can be achieved through various mechanisms, such as pH-dependent release, thermal triggering, or enzymatic degradation [54].

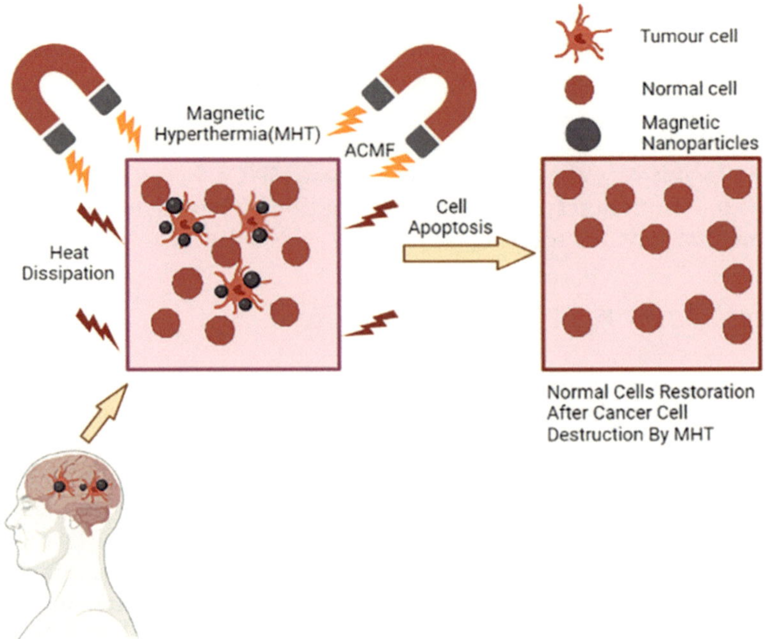

Figure 2.
Mechanism of magnetic nanocarrier for the treatment of glioma.

e. *Improved therapeutic effect*: The drugs or therapeutic agents released from the magnetic nanocarriers can exert their therapeutic effect on the glioma cells, inhibiting their growth or inducing apoptosis (programmed cell death) [55].

8. MNCs in brain tumor-targeted imaging and therapy

Magnetic nanoparticles (MNCs) have emerged as promising tools for brain tumor-targeted imaging and therapy. MNCs can be functionalized with specific ligands or antibodies that can target the nanoparticles to brain tumor cells, enabling precise localization and characterization of the tumor. MNCs can also be used to deliver therapeutic agents directly to the tumor site, increasing treatment efficacy while minimizing systemic toxicity [56].

Here are some of the ways that MNCs are being used for brain tumor-targeted imaging and therapy:

a. *Magnetic resonance imaging (MRI):* MNCs can be used as contrast agents for MRI. The unique magnetic properties of MNCs can generate strong signal changes in MRI, allowing for high-resolution imaging of the brain tumor. Targeted MNCs can be functionalized with specific ligands or antibodies that bind to receptors on the surface of brain tumor cells, enabling precise localization of the tumor [10].

b. *Magnetic hyperthermia:* MNCs can be used to generate heat through the application of an external magnetic field. This approach, known as magnetic hyperthermia, can induce tumor cell death and increase the efficacy of chemotherapy or radiation therapy. Targeted MNCs can be used to selectively heat tumor cells while sparing healthy tissue [57].

c. *Drug delivery:* MNCs can be used to deliver therapeutic agents directly to the brain tumor site. The MNCs can be functionalized with specific ligands or antibodies that target the tumor cells, allowing for precise delivery of the therapeutic agent to the tumor. This approach can increase the efficacy of the treatment while reducing systemic toxicity [10].

d. *Photodynamic therapy:* MNCs can also be used in combination with photodynamic therapy (PDT) to treat brain tumors. In this approach, targeted MNCs are functionalized with photosensitizing agents that generate reactive oxygen species (ROS) upon exposure to light. This approach can selectively induce cell death in tumor cells while sparing healthy tissue [58].

8.1 MNCs for hyperthermia

The basic principle of magnetic hyperthermia involves the application of an alternating magnetic field (AMF) to MNCs that have been localized to the tumor site. The AMF causes the MNCs to oscillate, generating heat through hysteresis losses in the surrounding tissue. The amount of heat generated by the MNCs can be controlled by adjusting the frequency and intensity of the applied AMF [59].

Here are some key factors that need to be considered when using MNCs for hyperthermia:

a. *Particle size and shape*: The size and shape of MNCs can affect their heating efficiency. Smaller particles tend to heat up more efficiently, but may also be more prone to aggregation. The shape of the particles can also affect their heating efficiency, with elongated particles often exhibiting higher heating efficiencies compared to spherical particles [60].

b. *Magnetic properties*: The magnetic properties of MNCs can also affect their heating efficiency. MNCs with high magnetic anisotropy exhibit larger hysteresis losses and higher heating efficiencies. However, the magnetic properties of MNCs can also affect their stability and biocompatibility [61].

c. *Targeting moieties*: Targeting moieties can be used to direct MNCs to the tumor site, allowing for selective heating of tumor cells while sparing normal tissue. Various targeting moieties, such as antibodies, peptides, and aptamers, have been investigated for use with MNCs [62].

d. *AMF parameters*: The frequency and intensity of the applied AMF can be adjusted to control the amount of heat generated by the MNCs. The optimal AMF parameters may vary depending on the size and magnetic properties of the MNCs, as well as the tumor microenvironment [63].

9. Recent advancements in MNCs based drug targeting

In a study published in the journal Nanoscale, researchers used magnetic nanoparticles loaded with doxorubicin (a chemotherapy drug) to treat glioma in mice. They found that the nanoparticles were able to cross the blood-brain barrier and accumulate in the tumor tissue, resulting in significant tumor growth inhibition [64].

Another study, published in the Journal of Controlled Release, investigated the use of magnetic nanoparticles to deliver small interfering RNA (siRNA) to glioma cells. The researchers found that the nanoparticles were able to effectively deliver siRNA, resulting in a significant knockdown of the targeted genes and inhibition of tumor growth [65].

In a study published in the journal Theranostics, researchers used magnetic nanoparticles in combination with alternating magnetic field hyperthermia to treat glioma in mice. They found that the combination therapy significantly inhibited tumor growth and prolonged the survival of the mice [66].

A recent review article published in the journal Frontiers in Pharmacology summarized the current state of research on magnetic nanoparticles for the treatment of glioma. The authors highlighted several promising approaches, including the use of magnetic nanoparticles for targeted drug delivery, hyperthermia, and multimodal therapy [67].

The creation of engineered MNCs that are able to be used as theranostic tools is progressing continuously. Although MNP platforms have made crucial progress, there are still technical knowledge gaps that prevent bench-to-bedside translation [68]. Before receiving regulatory clearance for human use, all MNP formulations should undergo thorough toxicological testing, taking into account the impact on various biological functions at the cellular & molecular level. Furthermore, there are restrictions with regard to magnetic targeting, in which the external magnetic field that is applied must be sufficiently powerful to capture the MNP-drug complexes at the location of choice [69]. Inducing and maintaining temperatures above the systemic temperature (37.5°C) in a specified target volume as well as achieving homogeneous heat distributions inside the intended organ are additional issues connected with hyperthermia-based treatment. Strong magnetic cores for MRI imaging, external magnets to assist with site-specific delivery of the MNCs to the targets, initiation of hyperthermia for temperature-triggered release of drugs, and a recognition layer for active targeting are all likely to be part of the MNCs of the future [70]. Finally, the therapeutic will likely be loaded to the coating material. Although the clinical uses of magnetic delivery of drugs are developing more slowly, the theranostic application, which will lead to personalized medicines, holds enormous potential. A ray of optimism exists for the clinic implementation of MNP-based theranostics thanks to the success of MRI and the development achieved so far in clinical trials [71].

In a different investigation, a formulation of zinc ferrite nanoparticles (ZFNP) with docetaxel (DTX) loaded on it was created and tested against C6 glioma cells. The findings suggest that ZFNP might be employed as a docetaxel nanodrug carrier for glioma cell delivery [72]. According to a recent review titled "Targeting to Brain Tumour: Nanocarrier-Based Drug Delivery Platforms, Opportunities, and Challenges," developments in the field of molecular neuroscience have actually revolutionized the use of nanotechnology-based approaches for the treatment of brain tumors that have spread to other parts of the body. In the upcoming years, it is anticipated that drug delivery systems based on nanocarriers will advance to new levels and significantly alter cancer research [73].

10. Challenges

While magnetic nanoparticles hold promise for the treatment of glioma, there are several challenges that need to be addressed before they can be widely used in clinical practice. Here are some of the main challenges:

a. *Blood-brain barrier (BBB) penetration:* The BBB is a major obstacle to the delivery of therapeutics to the brain. While magnetic nanoparticles can be functionalized to target glioma cells, they may still have difficulty crossing the BBB to reach the tumor site. Strategies to overcome this challenge include the use of focused ultrasound to temporarily disrupt the BBB and improve nanoparticle delivery.

b. *Specificity*: While magnetic nanoparticles can be targeted to glioma cells, it is important to ensure that they do not accumulate in healthy brain tissue. This requires the development of highly specific targeting strategies that can distinguish between glioma cells and normal brain cells.

c. *Toxicity*: Magnetic nanoparticles can potentially cause toxicity if they accumulate in non-target tissues or if they induce an immune response. It is important to carefully evaluate the safety of magnetic nanoparticles in preclinical studies before they can be used in humans.

d. *Clinical translation*: While there have been promising results in preclinical studies, it can be challenging to translate these findings into effective clinical therapies. The development of magnetic nanoparticle-based therapies for glioma will require extensive testing in clinical trials to evaluate their safety and efficacy.

e. *Cost*: Magnetic nanoparticle-based therapies can be expensive to develop and manufacture, which may limit their accessibility for patients.

f. One of the most difficult challenges is that the in *vivo* effects of diverse nanocarriers are sometimes considerably different from their in *vitro* activities. A significant gap in the *in vitro in vivo* correlation always exists for nanodrug carriers, making regulatory clearance difficult.

11. Conclusion

In conclusion, MNC-based drug targeting represents an emerging avenue for the treatment of glioma, providing a means to overcome the limitations associated with conventional glioma therapy. With continued advancements in nanotechnology, MNC-based strategies have the potential to revolutionize the field of glioma treatment, improving patient outcomes and quality of life. Moreover, the combination of MNCs with other therapeutic modalities, such as hyperthermia or photodynamic therapy, has shown synergistic effects in glioma treatment, further highlighting the potential of MNC-based approaches. However, in spite of MNCs holding tremendous promise, several challenges remain in their way of practical utilization, industrial scalability, or during technology transfer. Optimizing the design and synthesis of MNCs to achieve desirable properties, improving the understanding of MNC interactions with the BBB, checking industrial viability, and ensuring long-term in *vivo* safety and biocompatibility are some of the trending areas of ongoing research. Undoubtedly, with the successful scientific collaboration and increase in the volume of animal-related glioma experiments, some tangible outcome is expected in MNC-based glioma therapy in the near future.

Acknowledgements

The authors are very much grateful to Prof. Manoj Ranjan Nayak, President, Siksha 'O' Anusandhan (Deemed to be University) for providing the necessary facilities and encouragement.

Disclosure statement

The authors of the article have no conflict of interest to declare.

Author details

Bhabani Sankar Satapathy[1*], Jnanranjan Panda[2], Biswabhusan Biswal[1], Abhishek Mishra[1], Snigdha Pattnaik[1], Pralaya Kumar Sahoo[1] and Anshuman Gouda[3]

1 School of Pharmaceutical Sciences, Siksha 'O' Anusandhan University, Kalinganagar, Bhubaneswar, Odisha, India

2 Sri Sri University, Cuttack, Odisha, India

3 Royal College of Pharmacy and Health Sciences, Berhampur, Odisha, India

*Address all correspondence to: bhabanisatapathy@soa.ac.in

References

[1] Davis ME. Epidemiology and overview of gliomas. Seminars in Oncology Nursing. 2018;**34**(5):420-429. WB Saunders. DOI: 10.1016/j.soncn.2018.10.001

[2] Wiemels JL, Wiencke JK, Sison JD, Miike R, McMillan A, Wrensch M. History of allergies among adults with glioma and controls. International Journal of Cancer. 2002;**98**(4):609-615. DOI: 10.1002/ijc.10239

[3] Molinaro AM, Taylor JW, Wiencke JK, Wrensch MR. Genetic and molecular epidemiology of adult diffuse glioma. Nature Reviews Neurology. 2019;**15**(7):405-417. DOI: 10.1038/s41582-019-0220-2

[4] Gladson CL, Prayson RA, Liu WM. The pathobiology of glioma tumors. Annual Review of Pathology: Mechanisms of Disease. 2010;**5**:33-50. DOI: 10.1146/annurev-pathol-121808-102109

[5] Nuriya M, Shinotsuka T, Yasui M. Diffusion properties of molecules at the blood-brain interface: Potential contributions of astrocyte endfeet to diffusion barrier functions. Cerebral Cortex. 2013;**23**(9):2118-2126

[6] Fernandes C, Costa A, Osório L, Lago RC, Linhares P, Carvalho B, et al. Current Standards of Care in Glioblastoma Therapy. Brisbane, Australia: Exon Publications; 2017. pp. 197-241. DOI: 10.15586/codon.glioblastoma.2017.ch11

[7] Armstrong TS, Bishof AM, Brown PD, Klein M, Taphoorn MJ, Theodore-Oklota C. Determining priority signs and symptoms for use as clinical outcomes assessments in trials including patients with malignant gliomas: Panel 1 report. Neuro-Oncology. 2016;**18**(suppl_2):ii1-ii2. DOI: 10.1093/neuonc/nov267

[8] Bush NA, Chang SM, Berger MS. Current and future strategies for treatment of glioma. Neurosurgical Review. 2017;**40**:1-4. DOI: 10.1007/s10143-016-0709-8

[9] Carlsson SK, Brothers SP, Wahlestedt C. Emerging treatment strategies for glioblastoma multiforme. EMBO Molecular Medicine. 2014;**6**(11):1359-1370. DOI: 10.15252/emmm.201302627

[10] Sun C, Lee JS, Zhang M. Magnetic nanoparticles in MR imaging and drug delivery. Advanced Drug Delivery Reviews. 2008;**60**(11):1252-1265. DOI: 10.1016/j.addr.2008.03.018

[11] Kim DK, Dobson J. Nanomedicine for targeted drug delivery. Journal of Materials Chemistry. 2009;**19**(35):6294-6307. DOI: 10.1039/b902711b

[12] Mohseni M, Connell JJ, Payne C, Patrick PS, Baker R, Yu Y, et al. Scalable magnet geometries enhance tumour targeting of magnetic nano-carriers. Materials & Design. 2020;**191**:108610. DOI: 10.1016/j.matdes.2020.108610

[13] Li X, Tsibouklis J, Weng T, Zhang B, Yin G, Feng G, et al. Nano carriers for drug transport across the blood-brain barrier. Journal of Drug Targeting. 2017;**25**(1):17-28. DOI: 10.1080/1061186X.2016.1184272

[14] De Vries NA, Beijnen JH, Boogerd W, Van Tellingen O. Blood-brain barrier and chemotherapeutic treatment of brain tumors. Expert Review of

Neurotherapeutics. 2006;**6**(8):1199-1209. DOI: 10.1586/14737175.6.8.1199

[15] Kadry H, Noorani B, Cucullo L. A blood-brain barrier overview on structure, function, impairment, and biomarkers of integrity. Fluids and Barriers of the CNS. 2020;**17**(1):1-24. DOI: 10.1186/s12987-020-00230-3

[16] Engelhardt B, Sorokin L. The blood-brain and the blood–cerebrospinal fluid barriers: Function and dysfunction. Seminars in Immunopathology. 2009;**31**:497-511. Springer-Verlag. DOI: 10.1007/s00281-009-0177-0

[17] Pong S, Karmacharya R, Sofman M, Bishop JR, Lizano P. The role of brain microvascular endothelial cell and blood-brain barrier dysfunction in schizophrenia. Complex Psychiatry. 2020;**6**(1-2):30-46. DOI: 10.1159/000511552

[18] Furtado D, Björnmalm M, Ayton S, Bush AI, Kempe K, Caruso F. Overcoming the blood-brain barrier: The role of nanomaterials in treating neurological diseases. Advanced Materials. 2018;**30**(46):1801362. DOI: 10.1002/adma.201801362

[19] Thomsen MS, Routhe LJ, Moos T. The vascular basement membrane in the healthy and pathological brain. Journal of Cerebral Blood Flow & Metabolism. 2017;**37**(10):3300-3317. DOI: 10.1177/0271678X1772243

[20] Bhowmik A, Khan R, Ghosh MK. Blood brain barrier: A challenge for effectual therapy of brain tumors. BioMed Research International. 2015:1-20. DOI: 10.1155/2015/320941

[21] Abbott NJ. Astrocyte–endothelial interactions and blood–brain barrier permeability. Journal of Anatomy. 2002;**200**(5):523-534. DOI: 10.1046/j.1469-7580.2002.00047_13.x

[22] Galea I. The blood–brain barrier in systemic infection and inflammation. Cellular & Molecular Immunology. 2021;**18**(11):2489-2501. DOI: 10.1038/s41423-021-00757-x

[23] Greene C, Campbell M. Tight junction modulation of the blood brain barrier: CNS delivery of small molecules. Tissue Barriers. 2016;**4**(1):e1138017. DOI: 10.1080/21688370.2015.1138017

[24] Redzic Z. Molecular biology of the blood-brain and the blood-cerebrospinal fluid barriers: Similarities and differences. Fluids and Barriers of the CNS. 2011;**8**(1):1-25. Available from: http://www.fluidsbarrierscns.com/content/8/1/3

[25] Youdim MB, Edmondson D, Tipton KF. The therapeutic potential of monoamine oxidase inhibitors. Nature Reviews Neuroscience. 2006;**7**(4):295-309. DOI: 10.1038/nrn1883

[26] Motz CT, Kabat V, Saxena T, Bellamkonda RV, Zhu C. Neuromechanobiology: An expanding field driven by the force of greater focus. Advanced Healthcare Materials. 2021;**10**(19):2100102. DOI: 10.1002/adhm.202100102

[27] Baeten KM, Akassoglou K. Extracellular matrix and matrix receptors in blood–brain barrier formation and stroke. Developmental Neurobiology. 2011;**71**(11):1018-1039. DOI: 10.1002/dneu.20954

[28] Serlin Y, Shelef I, Knyazer B, Friedman A. Anatomy and physiology of the blood–brain barrier. Seminars in Cell & Developmental Biology. 2015;**38**:2-6. Academic Press. DOI: 10.1016/j.semcdb.2015.01.002

[29] Kumar R, Shin WS, Sunwoo K, Kim WY, Koo S, Bhuniya S, et al. Small conjugate-based theranostic agents: An encouraging approach for cancer therapy. Chemical Society Reviews. 2015;**44**(19):6670-6683. DOI: 10.1039/c5cs00224a

[30] Cheng Z, Li M, Dey R, Chen Y. Nanomaterials for cancer therapy: Current progress and perspectives. Journal of Hematology & Oncology. 2021;**14**(1):1-27. DOI: 10.1186/s13045-021-01096-0

[31] Dilnawaz F, Sahoo SK. Therapeutic approaches of magnetic nanoparticles for the central nervous system. Drug Discovery Today. 2015;**20**(10):1256-1264. DOI: 10.1016/j.drudis.2015.06.008

[32] Laquintana V, Trapani A, Denora N, Wang F, Gallo JM, Trapani G. New strategies to deliver anticancer drugs to brain tumors. Expert Opinion on Drug Delivery. 2009;**6**(10):1017-1032. DOI: 10.1517/17425240903167942

[33] Sathornsumetee S, Reardon DA, Desjardins A, Quinn JA, Vredenburgh JJ, Rich JN. Molecularly targeted therapy for malignant glioma. Cancer. 2007;**110**(1):13-24. DOI: 10.1002/cncr.22741

[34] Spandana KA, Bhaskaran M, Karri VR, Natarajan J. A comprehensive review of nano drug delivery system in the treatment of CNS disorders. Journal of Drug Delivery Science and Technology. 2020;**57**:101628. DOI: 10.1016/j.jddst.2020.101628

[35] Vangijzegem T, Stanicki D, Laurent S. Magnetic iron oxide nanoparticles for drug delivery: Applications and characteristics. Expert Opinion on Drug Delivery. 2019;**16**(1):69-78. DOI: 10.1080/17425247.2019.1554647

[36] Al-Jamal WT, Kostarelos K. Liposomes: From a clinically established drug delivery system to a nanoparticle platform for theranostic nanomedicine. Accounts of Chemical Research. 2011;**44**(10):1094-1104. DOI: 10.1021/ar200105p

[37] Ulbrich K, Hola K, Subr V, Bakandritsos A, Tucek J, Zboril R. Targeted drug delivery with polymers and magnetic nanoparticles: Covalent and noncovalent approaches, release control, and clinical studies. Chemical Reviews. 2016;**116**(9):5338-5431. DOI: 10.1021/acs.chemrev.5b00589

[38] Sun W, Mignani S, Shen M, Shi X. Dendrimer-based magnetic iron oxide nanoparticles: Their synthesis and biomedical applications. Drug Discovery Today. 2016;**21**(12):1873-1885. DOI: 10.1016/j.drudis.2016.06.028

[39] Thiruvengadathan R, Korampally V, Ghosh A, Chanda N, Gangopadhyay K, Gangopadhyay S. Nanomaterial processing using self-assembly-bottom-up chemical and biological approaches. Reports on Progress in Physics. 2013;**76**(6):066501. DOI: 10.1088/0034-4885/76/6/066501

[40] Ali A, Shah T, Ullah R, Zhou P, Guo M, Ovais M, et al. Review on recent progress in magnetic nanoparticles: Synthesis, characterization, and diverse applications. Frontiers in Chemistry. 2021;**9**:629054. DOI: 10.3389/fchem.2021.629054

[41] Semaltianos NG, Karczewski G. Laser synthesis of magnetic nanoparticles in liquids and application in the fabrication of polymer–nanoparticle composites. ACS Applied Nano Materials. 2021;**4**(7):6407-6440. DOI: 10.1021/acsanm.1c00715

[42] Ali A, Ovais M, Cui X, Rui Y, Chen C. Safety assessment of nanomaterials for antimicrobial applications. Chemical

Research in Toxicology [Internet]. 2020;**33**(5):1082-1109. DOI: 10.1021/acs.chemrestox.9b00519

[43] Tartaj P, del Puerto MM, Veintemillas-Verdaguer S, Gonzalez-Carreno T, Serna CJ. The preparation of magnetic nanoparticles for applications in biomedicine. Journal of Physics D: Applied Physics. 2003;**36**(13):R182. DOI: 10.1088/0022-3727/36/13/202

[44] Paswan SK, Kumar P, Singh RK, Shukla SK, Kumar L. Spinel ferrite magnetic nanoparticles: An alternative for wastewater treatment. In: Pollutants and Water Management: Resources, Strategies and Scarcity. New Jersey, USA: Wiley; 2021. pp. 273-305. DOI: 10.1002/9781119693635.ch11

[45] Mokhosi SR, Mdlalose W, Nhlapo A, Singh M. Advances in the synthesis and application of magnetic ferrite nanoparticles for cancer therapy. Pharmaceutics. 2022;**14**(5):937. DOI: 10.3390/pharmaceutics14050937

[46] Mollarasouli F, Zor E, Ozcelikay G, Ozkan SA. Magnetic nanoparticles in developing electrochemical sensors for pharmaceutical and biomedical applications. Talanta. 2021;**226**:122108. DOI: 10.1016/j.talanta.2021.122108

[47] Kale SN, Deore SL. Emulsion micro emulsion and nano emulsion: A review. Systematic Reviews in Pharmacy. 2017;**8**(1):39. DOI: 10.5530/srp.2017.1.8

[48] Dudchenko N, Pawar S, Perelshtein I, Fixler D. Magnetite nanoparticles: Synthesis and applications in optics and nanophotonics. Materials. 2022;**15**(7):2601. DOI: 10.3390/ma15072601

[49] Zha J, Roggendorf H. Advance material. In: Brinker CJ, Scherer GW, editors. Sol–Gel Science, The Physics and Chemistry of Sol–Gel Processing. Vol. 3. No. 10, xiv Boston: Academic Press; 1990. p. 908. bound—ISBN 0-12-134970-5. DOI: 10.1002/adma.19910031025

[50] Nair GM, Sajini T, Mathew B. Advanced green approaches for metal and metal oxide nanoparticles synthesis and their environmental applications. Talanta Open. 2022;**5**:100080. DOI: 10.1016/j.talo.2021.100080

[51] Liu HL, Hua MY, Yang HW, Huang CY, Chu PC, Wu JS, et al. Magnetic resonance monitoring of focused ultrasound/magnetic nanoparticle targeting delivery of therapeutic agents to the brain. Proceedings of the National Academy of Sciences. 2010;**107**(34):15205-15210. DOI: 10.1073/pnas.1003388107

[52] Barbu E, Molnàr É, Tsibouklis J, Górecki DC. The potential for nanoparticle-based drug delivery to the brain: Overcoming the blood–brain barrier. Expert Opinion on Drug Delivery. 2009;**6**(6):553-565. DOI: 10.1517/17425240902939143

[53] Hartl N, Adams F, Merkel OM. From adsorption to covalent bonding: Apolipoprotein E functionalization of polymeric nanoparticles for drug delivery across the blood–brain barrier. Advanced Therapeutics. 2021;**4**(1):2000092. DOI: 10.1002/adtp.202000092

[54] Navya PN, Kaphle A, Srinivas SP, Bhargava SK, Rotello VM, Daima HK. Current trends and challenges in cancer management and therapy using designer nanomaterials. Nano Convergence. 2019;**6**:1-30. DOI: 10.1186/s40580-019-0193-2

[55] Zhang Y, Xi K, Fu X, Sun H, Wang H, Yu D, et al. Versatile metal-phenolic network nanoparticles for multitargeted

combination therapy and magnetic resonance tracing in glioblastoma. Biomaterials. 2021;**278**:121163. DOI: 10.1016/j.biomaterials.2021.121163

[56] Parveen S, Misra R, Sahoo SK. Nanoparticles: A boon to drug delivery, therapeutics, diagnostics and imaging. Nanomedicine: Nanotechnology, Biology and Medicine. 2012;**8**(2):147-166. DOI: 10.1016/j.nano.2011.05.016

[57] Murase K, Takata H, Takeuchi Y, Saito S. Control of the temperature rise in magnetic hyperthermia with use of an external static magnetic field. Physica Medica. 2013;**29**(6):624-630. DOI: 10.1016/j.ejmp.2012.08.005

[58] Sarbadhikary P, George BP, Abrahamse H. Recent advances in photosensitizers as multifunctional theranostic agents for imaging-guided photodynamic therapy of cancer. Theranostics. 2021;**11**(18):9054. DOI: 10.7150/thno.62479

[59] Liu X, Zhang Y, Wang Y, Zhu W, Li G, Ma X, et al. Comprehensive understanding of magnetic hyperthermia for improving antitumor therapeutic efficacy. Theranostics. 2020;**10**(8):3793. DOI: 10.7150/thno.40805

[60] Obaidat IM, Issa B, Haik Y. Magnetic properties of magnetic nanoparticles for efficient hyperthermia. Nanomaterials. 2015;**5**(1):63-89. DOI: 10.3390/nano5010063

[61] Lanier OL, Korotych OI, Monsalve AG, Wable D, Savliwala S, Grooms NW, et al. Evaluation of magnetic nanoparticles for magnetic fluid hyperthermia. International Journal of Hyperthermia. 2019;**36**(1):686-700. DOI: 10.1080/02656736.2019.1628313

[62] Wadajkar AS, Menon JU, Kadapure T, Tran RT, Yang J, Nguyen KT. Design and application of magnetic-based theranostic nanoparticle systems. Recent Patents on Biomedical Engineering (Discontinued). 2013;**6**(1):47-57. DOI: 10.2174/1874764711306010007

[63] Gavilán H, Avugadda SK, Fernández-Cabada T, Soni N, Cassani M, Mai BT, et al. Magnetic nanoparticles and clusters for magnetic hyperthermia: Optimizing their heat performance and developing combinatorial therapies to tackle cancer. Chemical Society Reviews. 2021;**50**(20):11614-11667. DOI: 10.1039/d1cs00427a

[64] Norouzi M, Yathindranath V, Thliveris JA, Kopec BM, Siahaan TJ, Miller DW. Doxorubicin-loaded iron oxide nanoparticles for glioblastoma therapy: A combinational approach for enhanced delivery of nanoparticles. Scientific Reports. 2020;**10**(1):11292. DOI: 10.1038/s41598-020-68017-y

[65] Gandhi NS, Tekade RK, Chougule MB. Nanocarrier mediated delivery of siRNA/miRNA in combination with chemotherapeutic agents for cancer therapy: Current progress and advances. Journal of Controlled Release. 2014;**194**:238-256. DOI: 10.1016/j.jconrel.2014.09.001

[66] Rodrigues HF, Capistrano G, Bakuzis AF. In vivo magnetic nanoparticle hyperthermia: A review on preclinical studies, low-field nano-heaters, noninvasive thermometry and computer simulations for treatment planning. International Journal of Hyperthermia. 2020;**37**(3):76-99. DOI: 10.1080/02656736.2020.1800831

[67] Jain KK. A critical overview of targeted therapies for glioblastoma. Frontiers in Oncology. 2018;**8**:419. DOI: 10.3389/fonc.2018.00419

[68] Cole AJ, Yang VC, David AE. Cancer theranostics: The rise of targeted

magnetic nanoparticles. Trends in Biotechnology. 2011;**29**(7):323-332. DOI: 10.1016/j.tibtech.2011.03.001

[69] Gupta R, Xie H. Nanoparticles in daily life: Applications, toxicity and regulations. Journal of Environmental Pathology, Toxicology and Oncology. 2018;**37**(3):209-230. DOI: 10.1615/JEnvironPatholToxicolOncol.2018026009

[70] Kumar CS, Mohammad F. Magnetic nanomaterials for hyperthermia-based therapy and controlled drug delivery. Advanced Drug Delivery Reviews. 2011;**63**(9):789-808. DOI: 10.1016/j.addr.2011.03.008

[71] Siafaka PI, Okur NÜ, Karantas ID, Okur ME, Gündoğdu EA. Current update on nanoplatforms as therapeutic and diagnostic tools: A review for the materials used as nanotheranostics and imaging modalities. Asian Journal of Pharmaceutical Sciences. 2021;**16**(1):24-46. DOI: 10.1016/j.ajps.2020.03.003

[72] Panda J, Satapathy BS, Sarkar R, Tudu B. A zinc ferrite nanodrug carrier for delivery of docetaxel: Synthesis, characterization, and in vitro tests on C6 glioma cells. Journal of Microencapsulation. 2022;**39**(2):136-144. DOI: 10.1080/02652048.2022.2053757

[73] Kumar LA, Pattnaik G, Satapathy BS, Swapna S, Mohanty D. Targeting to brain tumor: Nanocarrier-based drug delivery platforms, opportunities, and challenges. Journal of Pharmacy & Bioallied Sciences. 2021;**13**(2):172. DOI: 10.4103/jpbs.JPBS_239_20

Section 2

4D MRI Glioma Tumor Classification

Chapter 5

Deep Learning for Computer-Aided Diagnosis (CAD) of Brain Diseases Four-Dimensional Magnetic Resonance Imaging (4D MRI Classification) from Glioma Tumor

Ismail Boukli Hacene and Zineb Aziza Elaouaber

Abstract

This work focuses on the utilization of Deep Learning and Convolutional Neural Networks (CNNs) for the accurate segmentation of a glioma tumor in brain magnetic resonance imaging (MRI) images. Specifically, we employed three distinct architectures using the labeled database BraTS2018 for training. To accomplish this, we utilized MATLAB 2019, which is compatible with Graphic Processing Unit (GPU) for enhanced performance. We have utilized various layers of a CNN to construct our architectures, including the convolutional layer, pooling layer, rectification layer, deconvolutional layer, and loss layer, to perform semantic segmentation. In addition, we compared the results obtained using the Dice coefficient. We show that the choice of epoch number has a great influence and a great importance for having the best results and giving better learning precision.

Keywords: deep learning, convolutional neural networks, segmentation, brain MRI images, glioma

1. Introduction

The growing mass of data, often volumetric, attracts the intention of the practitioner, to motivate the design of new automatic methods for the analysis and interpretation of images. Manual segmentation is an essential operation for any treatment and diagnosis.

To do this, the doctor must know exactly the changes that have occurred in the images, but this is not always obvious because of several artifacts and other peculiarities related to the specificities of the object to be segmented (the anatomy of the brain) and the magnetic resonance imaging (MRI) acquisition process making segmentation a laborious and difficult process. Thus, it is necessary to have diagnostic tools.

These support systems allow radiologists to have accurate information about the characteristics of the regions of interest sought.

The goal of our work is to develop a tool for segmenting the sections of brain MRI images of glioma patients that makes up about a third of the most common primary brain tumors, based on deep learning, aimed at helping neuro-anatomists and neuro-radiologists to identify the different forms of glioma lesions.

In this dissertation we develop three different convolutional neural network (CNN) models for glioma segmentation from four-dimensional magnetic resonance imaging (4D MRI) volumes, trying to increase the accuracy of the results by varying the parameters that make up the model.

2. Pathologies and brain tumors

A brain injury is a lesion that affects the brain. In general, it is a more or less extensive destruction of nerve tissue resulting in a deficit in perception, cognition, sensitivity, or motor skills depending on the role that the affected region played in the neurocognitive architecture.

After the age of 20, the human being loses thousands of neurons every day. This cellular degeneration is due to certain number of brain diseases such as brain tumors.

In our end-of-study project, we will focus on the detection of gliomas, which make up about a third of the most common primary brain tumors.

2.1 Glioma

Glioma is the most common form of a central nervous system (CNS) neoplasm that originates from glial cells in the brain [1]. These cells support the function of the other main type of brain cell: the neuron. Gliomas usually occur in the cerebral hemispheres of the brain, which are the largest and outermost parts of the brain that control many functions, including movement, speech, thinking, and emotions. However, they can also affect the brain stem, the lower part of the brain that controls functions such as breathing, blood pressure, heart rate, optic nerves, and the cerebellum, a part of the brain that deals with balance and other involuntary functions. These tumors can be benign or malignant. Generally, gliomas are classified into four grades. The fourth grade is the most aggressive type [2]: (1) Astrocytomas. (2). Ependymoma. (3). Glioblastoma. (4). Oligodendroglioma [3].

Headaches are the most common initial symptoms among glioma patients. These headaches are theoretically the result of tumor growth exerting a mass effect on the surrounding tissues. The mass effect, in turn, leads to pressure in the microvascularization and causes edema.

Depending on the tumor's location in the brain, the mass effect can result in specific signs of a brain tumor. For instance, frontal lobe tumors may exhibit behavioral changes, while dominant temporal lobe tumors may cause receptive speech problems.

Other symptoms related to mass effects include nausea, vomiting, and vision changes. Seizures are the second most common presenting symptoms. The pathophysiology of seizures is attributed to tumor irritation of the cerebral cortex, leading to focal or generalized seizures. Additional symptoms with gliomas may involve tingling sensations, weakness, difficulty walking, and in rare cases, patients may present in a comatose state due to tumor hemorrhage, leading to acute hernia syndrome [1].

Like most primary brain tumors, the exact cause of gliomas is unknown. But certain factors can increase the risk of developing a brain tumor. These risk factors include: age; radiation exposure, and family history of glioma [3].

3. State of the art

Currently, several researchers are interested in the segmentation and classification of cerebral glioma by deep learning from MRI images. Among them we mention:

Mahmoud Khaled Abd-Ellah et al. [4], introduced a new network structure for the accurate detection and classification of gliomatous tumors, using two parallel deep convolutional neural networks (PDCNNs). The PDCNN structure comprises local, global, fusion, and output paths, which are employed to classify input images into normal or glioma/tumor images, and further distinguish between HGG (high-grade gliomas) and LGG (low-grade gliomas). The local and global paths are utilized to extract local and global characteristics, respectively, and each path consists of seven convolutional layers with ReLU activation and 7 Max Pooling. In the local path, the first convolutional layer utilizes a 5 × 5-pixel filter size to capture local characteristics, while the global path's first convolutional layer uses a 12 × 12-pixel filter to extract global characteristics. After each convolutional layer in both paths, a Max Pooling is applied. Subsequently, the two paths are merged through a merging layer that establishes a cascading connection until the final output is reached. The merge path incorporates a normalization layer, followed by a rectified linear unit (ReLU) layer, and a fully connected layer connected to a dropout layer. The glioma classification process is facilitated on the output path using the Softmax function.

The performance of the proposed PDCNN was evaluated using the BraTS-2017 dataset, which comprises 600 normal two-dimensional (2D) images and 1200 abnormal 2D images. For the study, 1200 images were allocated to the training phase, 150 images to the validation phase, and 450 images to the test phase. The PDCNN structure achieved remarkable results in terms of accuracy, sensitivity, and specificity, with values of 97.44, 97.0, and 98.0%, respectively."

Jakub Nalepa et al. [5], presented data augmentation techniques applied to MRI images of brain tumors in the BraTS-2018 database. These techniques improve the generalization capabilities of deep neural networks (DNNs) by increasing the size of training sets and can be perceived as implicit regularization. These augmentation algorithms can be divided into the following main categories: algorithms exploiting various transformations of the original data, including affine image transformations (rotation, zoom, recalibration, symmetry according to horizontal and vertical axes, or translations), elastic transformations, transformations at the pixel level (the modification of the brightness of the image, the application of gamma correction...), and various approaches to generating artificial data.

Thus, the results obtained showed that the increase of data was essential in the most efficient algorithms, and form much deeper and more complex neural networks, also to face the problem of limited ground truth data.

Kaldera et al. [6] developed a CNN-based process for localization and segmentation of glioma tumors from grayscale MRI (2D sections) images.

This dataset consists of 3064 T1-weighted images with enhanced contrast, collected from 233 patients with three types of brain tumors: meningioma (708 slices), glioma (1426 slices), and pituitary tumor (930 slices). In glioma segmentation process, they selected 123 axial MRIs of separate brain tumors for training and testing. This process is based on a faster region-based convolutional neural network (R-CNN) architecture that consists of two types of network: the region proposal network (RPN) and the region-based convolutional neural network (R-CNN). This technique is very popular in terms of transfer learning because it can train a classifier on a smaller dataset. The R-CNN acts as a classifier and its accuracy is based on the performance of the RPN algorithm. The latter is developed by adding additional convolutional layers that produce an objectivity score at various points in the image. It also produces the regional boundaries of these regions of interest. In addition, the analysis shows that the proposed technique gave average detection accuracy, sensitivity, dice coefficient, and confidence level of 99.81, 87.72, 91.14 and 93.6%, respectively.

For glioma segmentation, Vinay Rao et al. [7] applied deep neural networks (DNNs) to the entire MRI base of BRATS-2015 brain tumors to classify each pixel accordingly. For the glioma category, the dataset includes images from each modality (T1, T1c, T2, and Flair), where the model captures information related to the neighborhood of each pixel in all modalities and combines them to form a multimodal representation. In this work 32x32 patches in the XY, YZ, and XZ planes around each pixel for each modality are extracted. These patches are introduced to the DNN for each modality in order to learn good representations for each pixel.

Each DNN is formed separately to classify a pixel among non-tumor, necrotizing, edema, non-improving, and improving pixels. Each of the DNNs is formed as follows: two layers of convolution each are followed by a Max Pooling, then two fully connected layers followed by the RELU function and the Softmax function are used to produce the output. Afterward, they used concatenation of representations of all modalities as characteristics to form a random forest classifier to classify pixels. This method achieved an accuracy of 67% on a test dataset.

4. Theory of deep learning

Deep learning is a collection of machine learning techniques that has facilitated significant advancements in artificial intelligence (AI) in recent years. In machine learning (ML), a program analyzes a dataset to derive rules that can be used to make predictions about new data.

Deep learning is built upon artificial neural networks (ANNs), which are analogously composed of thousands of units (neurons), each performing small, simple operations. The outputs of one layer of neurons serve as inputs for the next layer, and this process continues through multiple layers. The progress in deep learning has been made possible, particularly due to the increase in computational power and the development of large databases (big data).

4.1 Convolutional neural networks

Convolutional neural networks (CNNs) are currently the most efficient models for the classification, localization and segmentation of images, especially in the medical field. The CNNs have two distinct parts. As input, an image is provided as a pixel matrix. It has two dimensions for a grayscale image. The color is represented by a third dimension of depth 3 to represent the fundamental colors [Red, Green, and Blue].

The first part of a CNN is the convolutional part itself. It works as an extractor of image characteristics. An image is passed through a succession of filters, or convolution cores, creating new images called convolution maps. Some intermediate filters reduce the resolution of the image by a local maximum operation. In the end, the convolution maps are flattened and concatenated into a characteristic vector, called CNN code.

This CNN code (**Figure 1**) at the output of the convolutional part is then connected as the input of a second part, consisting of fully connected layers (multilayer

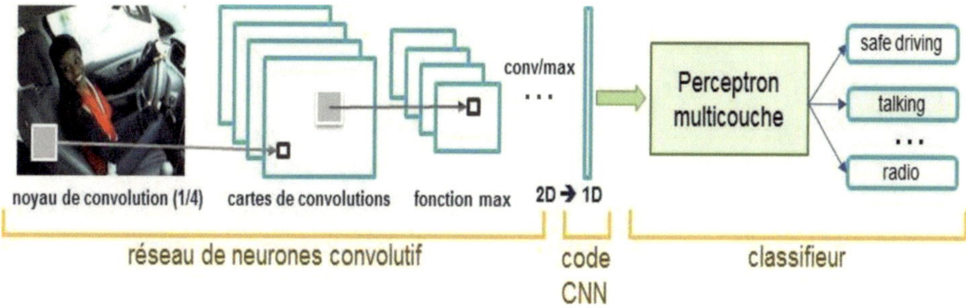

Figure 1.
Standard architecture of a CNN for image classification [8].

perceptron). The role of this part is to combine the characteristics of the CNN code to generate the output.

The output is the last layer with one neuron per category. The numerical values obtained are generally normalized between 0 and 1, of sum 1, to produce a probability distribution over the categories [8].

4.2 The most used deep learning segmentation models

4.2.1 Unet

U-Net is a model derived from the traditional convolutional neural network, specifically developed for biomedical image segmentation. It facilitates localization and segmentation by performing pixelwise classification, ensuring that the input and output share the same size. This renowned U-shaped model (**Figure 2**) is symmetrical and comprises two main parts:

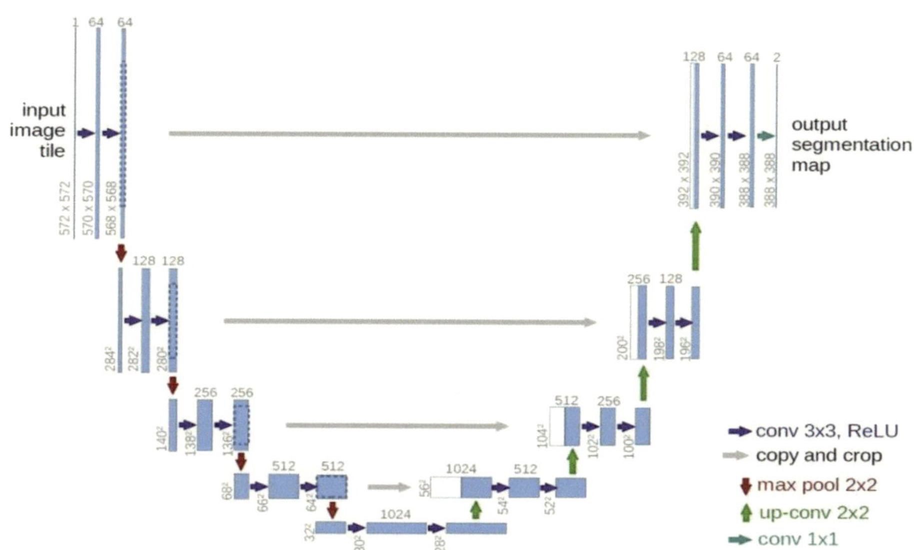

Figure 2.
The architecture of the Unet model [9].

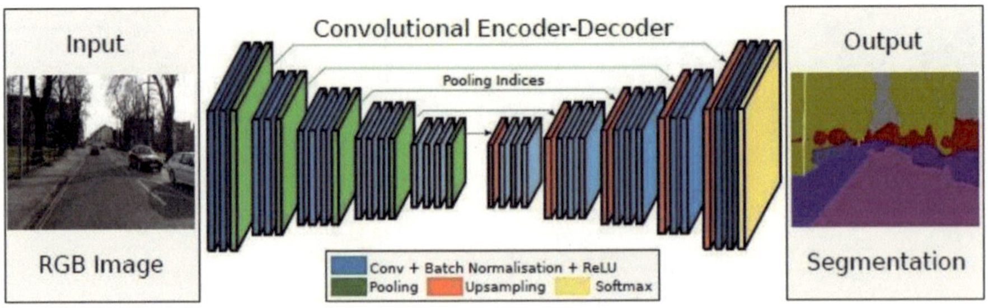

Figure 3.
The segmentation architecture by SegNet [12].

The left part, called the contraction path, consists of the general convolutional process, which involves multiple contraction blocks. Each block takes an input, applies two layers of 3x3 convolutions, followed by a RELU function, and Max Pooling (2x2). The number of filters or feature mappings doubles after each block, enabling the architecture to effectively learn complex structures [10].

The right part is the expansive path, consisting of transposed 2D convolutional layers. The number of expansion blocks matches the number of contraction blocks. Unet has the capability to perform precise image localization by predicting each pixel in the image individually [9].

4.2.2 SegNet

The SegNet model strikes a satisfactory balance between classification accuracy and computation time. Its symmetrical architecture allows for precise placement of abstract features in their correct spatial locations.

SegNet adopts an encoder-decoder architecture based on the convolutional layers of the VGG-16 model, which consists of 16 convolutional layers and is particularly attractive due to its uniform architecture [11]. The encoder is a series of convolutional layers followed by batch normalization (BN) and nonlinear activation functions (ReLU). Each block of two or three convolutions is subsequently followed by a subsampling layer (pooling) with a non-equal stride. The decoder is a mirror image of the encoder and possesses the same number of convolutions and blocks [12]. **Figure 3** shows the architecture of the SegNet model:

5. Experimental results

Gliomas are brain tumors caused by the abnormal proliferation of glial cells in the central nervous system. These tumors make up about one-third of the most common primary brain tumors. Indeed, the interest in glioma detection has increased with the development of imaging and computing power. In this chapter, we focus on glioma segmentation from MRI images.

In this part, we will present the hardware resources, the software used as well as the database used. Then, we will present the different architectures proposed. Then we will make a comparative study between the different methods used to improve the performance of a model in terms of time or efficiency. We will conclude with a discussion of the results achieved.

5.1 The database

Several brain MRI databases have been published in the literature, we have chosen the BraTS database named Task01_BrainTumour that was carried out in 2018 [13], which contains three folders: imagesTr, imagesTs, and labelsTr. The BraTS dataset is a collection of MRI scans focused on brain tumors, particularly gliomas, which are the most prevalent primary brain malignancies. This dataset comprises 750 4-D volumes, with each volume representing a stack of three-dimensional (3D) images in nifti format (.nii). The size of each 4D volume is (240 x 240 x 155 x 4), where the first three dimensions correspond to the height, width, and depth of a 3D volumetric image. The fourth dimension corresponds to distinct scanning modalities, such as "FLAIR," "T1w," "t1gd," and "T2w". The dataset is divided into 484 training volumes with voxel labels and 266 unlabeled test volumes. **Figure 4** shows a labeled 4D volume of the BraTS database.

5.2 Materials and methods

Several open source frameworks are available in the literature; we have chosen to work with the MATLAB R2019b language, which is easy to use.

Deep learning indeed requires substantial computational resources, and the availability of specialized resources like GPUs significantly impacts the user experience. Without these resources, the learning process can become excessively time-consuming, leading to longer training times and slower progress in learning from mistakes, which can be discouraging for users. Having access to powerful hardware accelerators like GPUs allows for faster training and more efficient learning, leading to a more positive and productive user experience. The experiments were all carried out on a machine that offers acceptable performance, the characteristics of which are as follows:

- Processor: AMD Ryzen threadripper 1950X 16-Core Processor 3.40 GHz.
- Installed memory (random access memory (RAM)): 16.0 GB.

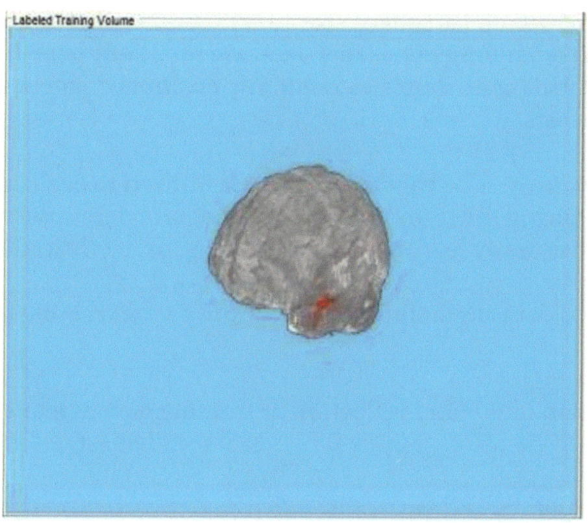

Figure 4.
Examples of a labeled training volume.

- 1 TB hard drive.
- System type: Windows 10 operating system, 64-bit, x64 processor.

5.3 Methods developed

The segmentation of medical images plays a major role in image processing and diagnostic aid, especially in the case of brain diseases. Among these diseases, there are primary brain tumors, where gliomas are the most common and have a poor prognosis. So, in this work we present a technique of segmentation of gliomas from 4D MRI volumes using deep learning.

5.3.1 Preprocessing of data

The test volumes do not have labels, so we did not use the test data. Instead, we divided the 484 learning volumes into three independent sets that are used for learning, validation, and testing. Next, we preprocessed the training and validation data to train the CNN network more efficiently. The data preprocessing involves several essential operations:

- *Cropping:* The data are cropped to focus on the brain and tumor region, reducing the dataset size while preserving crucial information in each MRI volume and its corresponding labels.
- *Normalization:* Each modality of every volume is normalized independently by subtracting the mean and dividing by the standard deviation of the cropped brain region.
- *Dataset split:* The 484 learning volumes are divided into 400 for training, 29 for validation, and 55 for testing purposes.
- *Random patch creation*: Patches of size 132x132x132x4, containing both the image and corresponding pixel label data, are randomly generated. Each pair of volumes and labels contributes 16 randomly positioned patches to the training and validation sets.
- *Validation data usage*: The validation data are utilized to evaluate the network's performance during the training process. It helps to determine whether the network is consistently learning, underlearning, or overlearning over time.

Next, we applied data augmentation operations to the training and validation data using:

- Random rotation of 90° and reflection of training data to make training more robust.
- Flipping horizontally and vertically.
- Cropping of response patches to network output size, 44 × 44 × 44 voxels.

5.3.2 Architecture of our network

In this part we proposed three different CNN architectures to perform binary semantic segmentation of brain tumors in MRI volumes, where each voxel is labeled as tumor or background.

5.3.2.1 First architecture (CNN 1)

As a first attempt, we started by forming a convolutional neural network of the most classic. This network consists of two convolutional layers each of which is followed by the ReLU activation function and a max pooling layer, then a deconvolutional layer is used to retrieve the size of the original input. Finally, the Softmax function is applied to produce the output. In this network, the voxel classification layer uses the Dice coefficient (allows the measurement of similarity in the labeled image and the resulting image) as the loss function to mitigate the problem of class imbalance in semantic segmentation problems.

The input volume, which has a size of 132x132x132x4, first moves to the first convolution layer. This layer is composed of 16 filters of size 3x3, followed by the RELU function that forces neurons to return positive values, and then we applied the Max Pooling to reduce the size of the image. This layer is composed of 16 filters of size 3x3, followed by the RELU function that forces neurons to return positive values, and then we applied the Max Pooling to reduce the size of the image. The second convolution layer consists of 32 filters of size 3x3, followed by a RELU and Max Pooling.

Then, we used a deconvolutional layer with seven size filters (2 × 2) in order to retrieve the original representation of our characteristics map and submit it to the last layer: Softmax.

The architecture of the first CNN formed is summarized in **Figure 5**.
As learning options we have chosen: Optimiseur = Adam;MiniBatchSize = 1,Max Epochs = 10,InitialLearnRate = 5e-4, LearnRateSchedule = piecewise,

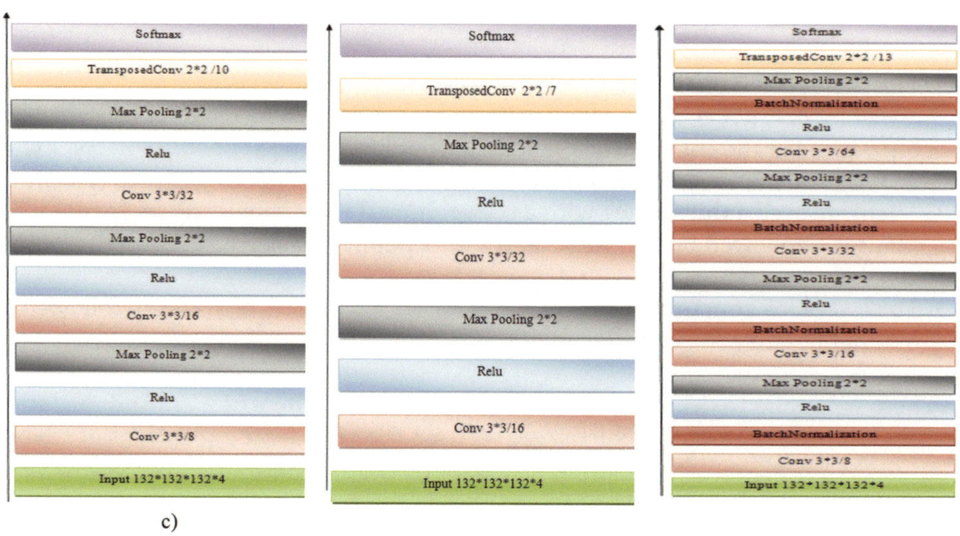

Figure 5.
Different architecture CNN formed. (a) The first CNN1; (b) the second CNN2; (c) the third CNN3 formed.

LearnRateDropPeriod = 5,LearnRateDropFactor = 0.95,ValidationFrequency = 400,ExecutionEnvironment = GPU.

5.3.2.2 Second architecture (CNN2)

The architecture depicted in **Figure 5** consists of three convolutional layers, each followed by the RELU function, a Max Pooling, and ultimately, a deconvolution layer. The Softmax function is then applied to generate the output. This network also uses the Dice coefficient as a loss function to classify voxels as tumors or backgrounds.

This time the input volume first passes through the first convolution layer. This layer is composed of 8 filters of size 3 × 3, followed by the RELU function and a Max Pooling of size (2 × 2). After applying the first convolutional layer with eight filters of size 3 × 3, the output of this layer is fed into the input of the second convolutional layer, which consists of 16 filters of size 3 × 3. The RELU activation function and a Max Pooling are then applied.

A third convolutional layer with 32 filters (3 × 3) was employed, followed by RELU activation and Max Pooling. Subsequently, a deconvolutional layer with 10 filters (2 × 2) was applied, and the architecture concluded with a Softmax layer.

In this case, we used the same CNN 1 learning options except the number of Epochs: Max Epochs = 50.

5.3.2.3 Third architecture (CNN3)

This third architecture, is composed of 4 convolutional layers with a different number of filters, each which is followed by a normalization layer (BN), the ReLU function and a Max pooling layer, then a deconvolution layer is used. Finally, the Softmax function is applied to produce the output. This network also uses the Dice coefficient as a loss function.

This time the input volume passes through four convolution blocks consisting of the following:

- The first block contains a convolution layer with eight filters of size 3x3, followed by BN, ReLU, and a Max pooling of size (2 × 2). The result of this block is introduced at the entrance of the second which contains a convolution layer with 16 filters of size 3x3, followed by BN, ReLU, and a Max pooling of size (2 × 2). Then, we used a third block with a convolutional layer consisting of 32 filters of size 3 × 3, followed by BN, ReLU and a Max pooling of size (2 × 2).

- The last block contains a convolution layer with 64 filters of size 3x3, followed by BN, ReLU, and a Max pooling of size (2 × 2).

Then, we applied a deconvolutional layer with 13 size filters (2 × 2). And the last layer was a Softmax. In this architecture, we used the same learning options of CNN 1.

5.4 Outcomes and discussion

During our experiments, we created three architectures where we applied the learning options by training the network using Adam's optimization solver and specifying the parameters using the "Training Options" function. These options are used to monitor the progress of the network's training. The initial learning rate is set at 5e-4, and then, it is adjusted regularly according to the MiniBatchSize.

In order to show the results obtained for these architectures, we illustrate in the following the results in terms of accuracy and error for each of the architectures.

5.4.1 First CNN

During training, the processor took 140.8 min to do 8000 iterations (finish training) with an error rate of 0.000475 and an accuracy of 99.08%.

Figure 6 shows the training progress of the CNN1 where the blue plot represents the training accuracy and the red plot represents the training loss.

Figure 7 shows the result of the semantic segmentation of gliomas by CNN1, where the tumors appear in red, the brain in gray, and the background in blue.

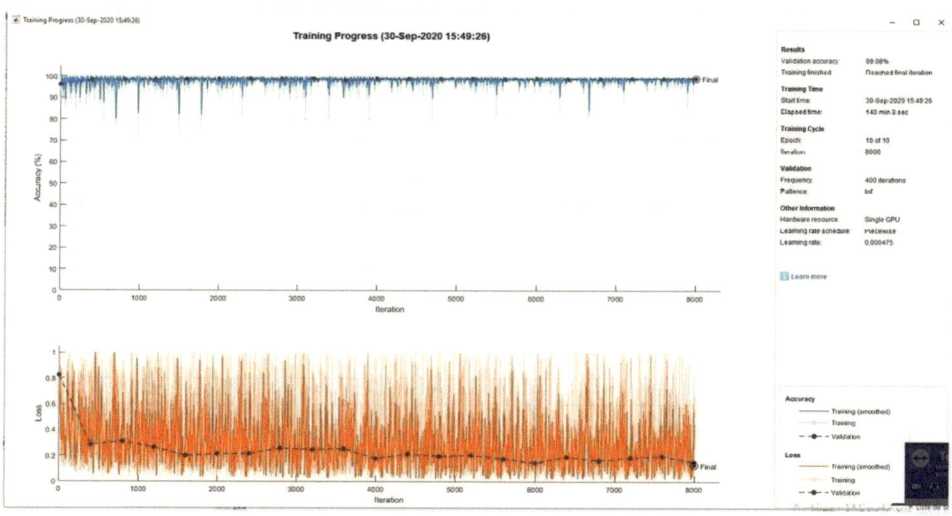

Figure 6.
Final progression of learning CNN1.

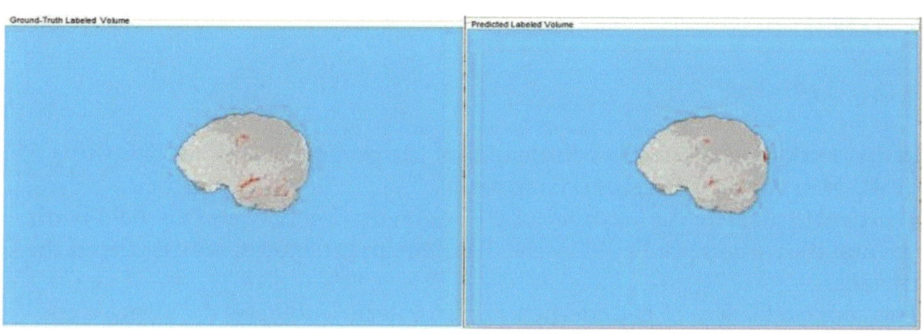

(a) (b)

Figure 7.
Segmentation result using CNN1; (a) field truth image; (b) predidated image.

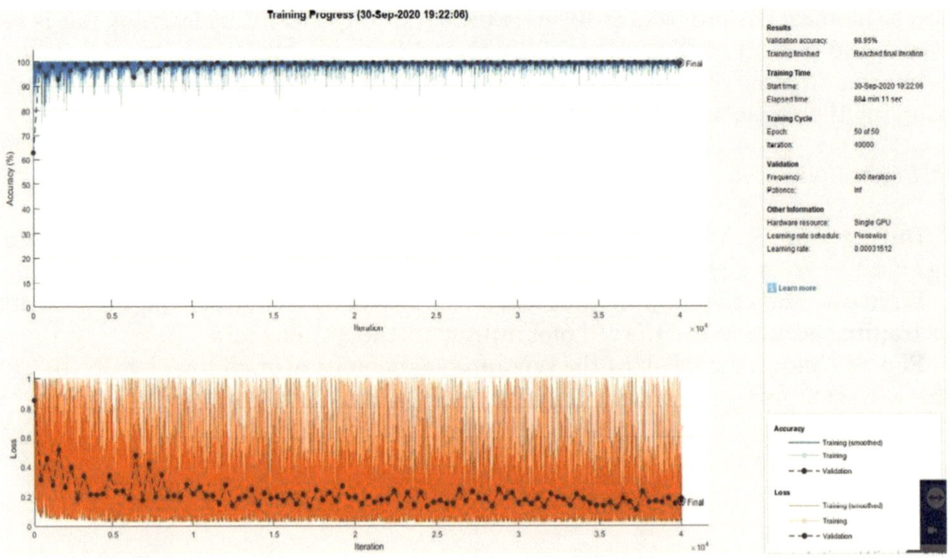

Figure 8.
Final progression of CNN2 learning.

5.4.2 Second CNN

We launched a learning of the second CNN. The processor took 884.11 min for 40,000 iterations with an error rate of 0.00031512 and an accuracy of 98.08%.

Figure 8 shows the training progress of the CN2.

Figure 9 below shows the result of the semantic segmentation of gliomas using CNN2.

5.4.3 Third CNN

Learning the third CNN took 314.03 minutes to complete 8000 iterations with an error rate of 0.000475 and an accuracy of 99.03%. **Figure 10** shows the training progress of the CNN3.

Figure 11 below shows the result of semantic segmentation of gliomas using CNN3 from 4D MRI volumes.

5.4.4 Dice coefficient

In this work, we tested the performance of the proposed CNN models using 55 image 4D MRI volumes from our database.

In order to calculate the accuracy of the segmentation between the field truth images and the images predicted by the different architectures, we calculated the Dice coefficient.

The Dice coefficient or the coefficient of similarity indicates the positive correlation between two images, it varies between 0 and 1, where 1 means the greatest similarity between prediction and truth.

Table 1 below shows the comparison between the different architectures used for glioma segmentation in terms of the Dice coefficient.

DOI: http://dx.doi.org/10.5772/intechopen.1002546

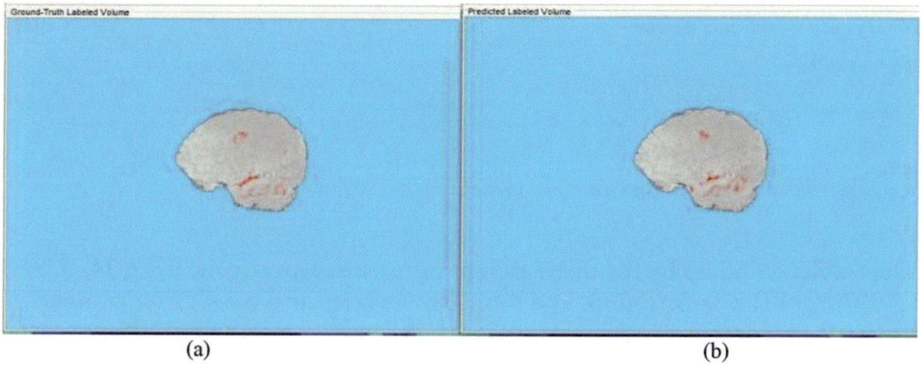

Figure 9.
Segmentation result using CNN2; (a) field truth image; (b) predidated image.

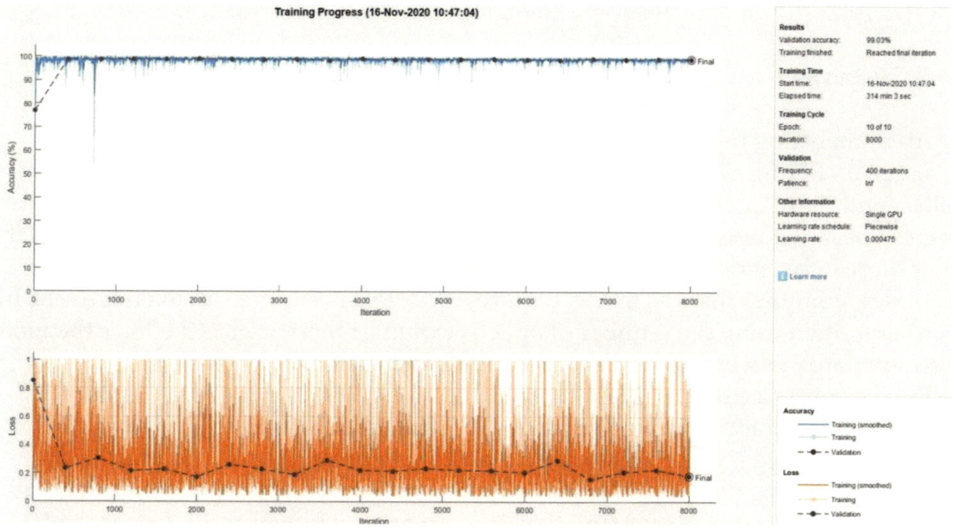

Figure 10.
Final progression of CNN3 learning.

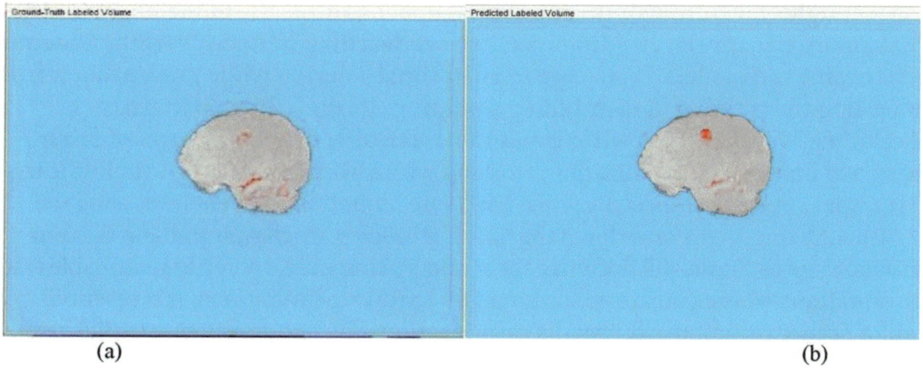

Figure 11.
Segmentation result using CNN3; (a) field truth image; (b) predidated image.

Architecture Coefficient de Dice	CNN1	CNN2	CNN3
For the substance	0.99834	0.99821	0.99797
For the tumor	0.83898	0.84799	0.79892

Table 1.
Coefficient de Dice obtenu par les différentes architectures.

The results obtained by the three architectures are respectively, 0.99834, 0.99821, and 0.99797 for the background, and 0.83898, 0.84799, and 0.79892 for tumors.

Thus, the results obtained are satisfactory and encouraging. The performance of the model can be enhanced by employing deeper and more complex architectures. Additionally, increasing the number of epochs and adjusting the MiniBatchSize, along with modifying the learning options, can also lead to improved results. These adjustments allow the model to learn more effectively and extract more intricate features from the data, ultimately enhancing its overall performance.

5.4.5 Comparison

After analyzing the results obtained, we note the following remarks:

Based on **Figures 7**, **9** and **11** information was previously featured in the CNN1, CNN2, and CNN3 architectures. The accuracy of learning generally improves with an increase in the number of epochs. This indicates that with each epoch, the model gains more information and refines its understanding of the data. If the accuracy decreases, it implies that the model requires more information to learn effectively. In such cases, increasing the number of epochs would be beneficial as it allows the model to accumulate more knowledge and enhance its performance.

Furthermore, as the number of epochs increases, the learning error tends to decrease. This reduction in error signifies that the model is converging toward a better solution and is becoming more proficient at the given task with each epoch. Therefore, training the model for more epochs can lead to better generalization and improved performance. So we find that in our work, architecture 2 is better than architecture 1 and architecture 3.

Also, the deeper the architecture, the better and more accurate the test result. Absolutely, the number of epochs and MiniBatchSize are crucial parameters in the learning process, and finding the right balance is essential for model performance.

As you rightly mentioned, the number of epochs allows the model to learn from the data more effectively, avoiding issues of overlearning or underlearning. Adequate epochs enable the model to converge to an optimal solution while preventing it from memorizing the training data or failing to capture its underlying patterns.

Regarding MiniBatchSize, while larger values can offer benefits in terms of faster training and improved generalization, working with a MiniBatchSize of 1 (online learning) is a valid approach, especially when hardware limitations prevent increasing the size. Although this might slow down the training process, stochastic gradient descent (MiniBatchSize of 1) can still optimize the model's parameters and yield reasonable results.

In situations where you are constrained by hardware limitations, it is essential to explore other techniques for model optimization. You can consider learning rate schedules, early stopping, and regularization to improve convergence and prevent overfitting. Additionally, exploring more computationally efficient model architectures can help work within the hardware capacity while achieving meaningful outcomes.

Remember, in practical applications, the balance between available resources and desired results often plays a crucial role, and many successful models can be built and trained with limited hardware settings. Adaptability and innovation in model design and optimization are key to obtaining satisfactory performance under such constraints.

6. Conclusion

The segmentation of medical images remains a very broad field of research. In the context of brain imaging, the goals of segmentation of brain MRI images are indeed multiple: help with diagnosis, monitoring of the evolution of the patient's condition, clinical test... etc.

The focus of our work is on the semantic segmentation of gliomas which are among the most common primary brain tumors, from magnetic resonance imaging (MRI) using convolutional neural networks (CNNs) that have shown its performance in recent years.

We have developed in this end-of-study project three different CNN architectures for the segmentation of gliomas from 4D MRI volumes inspired by an example of segmentation provided by MATLAB 2019. In the training phase, the use of a CPU makes the execution time too expensive. In order to solve this problem, it is necessary to use deep convolutional neural networks deployed on a GPU instead of a CPU.

To carry out our segmentation work, we used the BraTS database carried out in 2018, to learn the models and carried out the validations and testing part.

Network parameters are difficult to define *a priori*. That's why we have defined different models with different architectures to achieve better results in terms of accuracy and error.

The results found are satisfactory (a Dice coefficient for tumors of 83.8, 84.7 and 79.89% for the three architectures CNN1, CNN2 and CNN3, respectively), which allowed us to say that the use of semantic segmentation methods (deep learning) allows us to give better segmentation results.

Several perspectives can be envisaged in the extension of this dissertation, we can quote:

- Test other larger databases, and use deeper architectures like Unet and SegNet.
- Develop a tumor segmentation architecture based on 2D images.

Author details

Ismail Boukli Hacene* and Zineb Aziza Elaouaber
Research Biomedical Laboratory, Technology Faculty, Department of Biomedical Engineering, University Tlemcen, Algeria

*Address all correspondence to: ismaill80@yahoo.fr

References

[1] Mesfin FB, Al-Dhahir MA. Glioma. Treasure Island (FL): StatPearls Publishing; 2023

[2] Spinazzi EF, Argenziano MG, Upadhyayula PS, Banu MA, Neira JA, DMO H, et al. Chronic convection-enhanced delivery of topotecan for patients with recurrent glioblastoma: A first-in-patient, single-Centre, single-arm, phase 1b trial. The Lancet Oncology. 2022;**23**(11):1409-1418. DOI: 10.1016/S1470-2045(22)00599-X. Epub 2022 Oct 13

[3] Louis DN, et al. Classification and pathologic diagnosis of gliomas, glioneuronal tumors and neuronal tumors. Available from: https://www.uptodate.com/contents/search [Accessed: June 10, 2022].

[4] Abd-Ellah MK, Awad AI, Hamed HFA, Khalaf AAM. Parallel deep CNN structure for glioma detection and classification via brain MRI images. In: 2019 31st International Conference on Microelectronics (ICM), Cairo, Egypt. 2019. pp. 304-307. DOI: 10.1109/ICM48031.2019.9021872

[5] Nalepa J, Marcinkiewicz M, Kawulok M. Data augmentation for brain-tumor segmentation: A review. Frontiers in Computational Neuroscience. 2019;**13**:83. DOI: 10.3389/fncom.2019.00083

[6] Kaldera HNTK, Gunasekara SR, Dissanayake MB. MRI based glioma segmentation using deep learning algorithms. In: 2019 International Research Conference on Smart Computing and Systems Engineering (SCSE), Colombo, Sri Lanka. 2019. pp. 51-56. DOI: 10.23919/SCSE.2019.8842668

[7] Madhupriya G, Guru NM, Praveen S, Nivetha B. Brain tumor segmentation with deep learning technique. In: 2019 3rd International Conference on Trends in Electronics and Informatics (ICOEI), Tirunelveli, India. 2019. pp. 758-763. DOI: 10.1109/ICOEI.2019.8862575

[8] Mokri Mohammed Zakaria. Image Classification with Convolutional Neural Networks [thesis]. Algeria: Abou Bakr Belkaïd University of Tlemcen; 2017. Available from: http://dspace.univ-tlemcen.dz/bitstream/112/12235/1/Classification-des-images-avec-les-reseaux-de-neurones.pdf

[9] Krizhevsky A, Sutskever I, Hinton GE. ImageNet classification with deep convolutional neural networks. Communications of the ACM. Jun 2017;**60**(6):84-90. DOI: 10.1145/3065386

[10] Available from: https://datascientest.com/convolutional-neural-network [Accessed: June 2, 2022]

[11] Graham, Benjamin, Fractional Max-Pooling.Dept of Statistics, Dept of Statistics, University of Warwick, UK, Under review as a conference paper at ICLR 2015. Available from: https://arxiv.org/abs/1412.6071 [Accessed: June 2, 2022]

[12] Mohammed B, Brahim B. Deep Learning for Image Classification and Content-Based Image Retrieval [Online]. Kasdi Merbah University of Ouargla; 2016-2017. Available from: https://dspace.univ-ouargla.dz/jspui/bitstream/123456789/17195/1/Boughaba_Boukhris.pdf [Accessed: June 03, 2022]

[13] Bakas S, Reyes M, Jakab A, Bauer S, Rempfler M, Crimi A, et al. Identifying the best machine learning algorithms for brain tumor segmentation, progression assessment, and overall survival prediction in the BRATS challenge. arXiv. 2018